CORE
PERFORMANCE
ENDURANCE

INCREASE YOUR PERFORMANCE AND AVOID INJURIES

CORE
PERFORMANCE
ENDURANCE

**A NEW FITNESS AND NUTRITION PROGRAM
THAT REVOLUTIONIZES THE WAY YOU TRAIN
FOR ENDURANCE SPORTS**

MARK VERSTEGEN
AND PETE WILLIAMS

FOREWORD BY JESSI STENSLAND, Champion Triathlete

RODALE

Rodale books may be purchased for business or promotional use or for special sales. For information, please write to: Special Markets Department, Rodale Inc., 733 Third Avenue, New York, NY 10017.

Printed in the United States of America
Rodale Inc. makes every effort to use acid-free ⊛, recycled paper ♲.

Illustration on page 73 by Sandy Freeman
Photographs by David Zickl
Book design by Susan Eugster

Library of Congress Cataloging-in-Publication Data

Verstegen, Mark, date
   Core performance endurance : a new fitness and nutrition program that revolutionizes the way you train for endurance sports / by Mark Verstegen and Pete Williams ; foreword by Jessi Stensland.
     p.   cm.
   Includes index.
   ISBN-13 978–1–59486–352–3 hardcover
   ISBN-10 1–59486–352–0 hardcover
   1. Endurance sports. 2. Physical fitness. 3. Nutrition. I. Williams, Pete, date II. Title.
GV749.5.V47 2006
613.7'1—dc22   2006029367

Distributed to the trade by Holtzbrinck Publishers

2 4 6 8 10 9 7 5 3 1 hardcover

RODALE
LIVE YOUR WHOLE LIFE™

We inspire and enable people to improve their lives and the world around them
For more of our products visit **rodalestore.com** or call 800-848-4735

CONTENTS

Foreword: By Jessi Stensland vii

Introduction: The Endurance Paradigm Shift xiii

PART 1
THE CORE ENDURANCE MINDSET

1: A Call to Change 3

2: Self-Evaluation 11

PART 2
CORE ENDURANCE MOVEMENT

3: Building Your Pillar 25

4: Power Endurance 35

5: Energy System Development 43

6: Regeneration 51

PART 3
CORE ENDURANCE NUTRITION

7: Eat to Perform 61

8: Timing Is Everything 85

PART 4
THE CORE ENDURANCE WORKOUT

9: The Core Endurance Workout:
An Introduction 105

10: Core Movements 117

FAQs 215

Afterword 221

Acknowledgments 227

Index 229

About the Authors 237

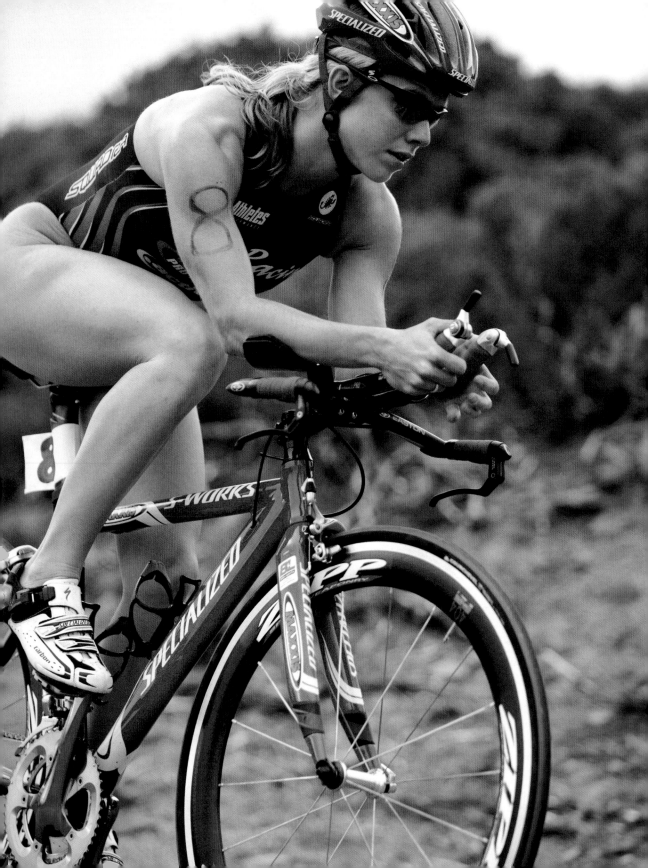

FOREWORD

By Jessi Stensland

Professional Triathlete

Mastering endurance sports, like any challenge, takes time and energy. Endurance athletes are not drawn to compete because their sports are going to be easy, of course. It's the feeling of accomplishment, of meeting challenges and reaching goals, that motivates us. We *endure.*

I've been competing in endurance sports for more than 20 years, 6 as a professional triathlete. I've always believed that I've had the potential to be among the best athletes in the world. There was a time, however, when I began to doubt that I could fulfill that potential. It's not that I lost faith in myself; I knew I was capable. My body simply no longer was able to do what I asked of it. It seemed so beat-up from years of training and racing that I wasn't sure it was possible to reverse the damage.

I became frustrated and even thought my career was over. Thankfully, I didn't give up. I searched for answers and a greater understanding of my body and its capabilities. Mark Verstegen's Core Performance system literally saved my career and has propelled me to heights I never thought imaginable.

Core Performance Endurance is much more than a training program. From the beginning, you will develop a performance mindset and learn exercises that incorporate strength, power, stability, and flexibility. Mark will teach you how each of these elements complements every endurance activity and is vital to performance, whether you're a recreational runner or someone whose goal is competing in the Ironman Triathlon. It won't take long for you to feel stronger and more stable, to have greater power and flexibility, to recover faster. Best of all, you'll start having more fun.

Once I started working with Mark, it wasn't long before I again looked forward to many more years of endurance sports competition. I saw immediate improvements. Now, after more than 3 years following the program, I continue to see improvement in every workout and race. Even more rewarding is that I have an extra spring in my step. I stand taller and run taller. I'm more confident on and off the racecourse. The physical benefits are endless. I now have the confidence to take on challenge after challenge, and I possess a body that has the ability to endure in my athletic endeavors and in day-to-day life. Since embarking on this program, I've felt nothing short of invincible.

Still, being an endurance athlete has its ups and downs. We're tough, always fighting through pain, at times pushing through it to the point of injury. We tend to think of training in terms of long hours and how many miles we can pack into the precious time we have. We're so busy juggling commitments that we often neglect our bodies, the very vehicles that we're using to accomplish our endurance goals. *Core Performance Endurance* provides simple ways to maintain and improve our bodies that can be seamlessly incorporated into training.

Don't be surprised to read things in this book that fly in the face of conventional wisdom. Endurance athletes long have been told to utilize weight training only in the off-season, and even then to perform only low-weight and high-rep routines. If you think about it, we're already doing low-weight, high-rep routines with each step running and each stroke in the water or on the bicycle. With *Core Performance Endurance* you will do the opposite, performing a lower number of reps with higher weight in order to gain strength and power. You'll also train your neuromuscular system, giving you better control over your body and your effort.

You'll significantly decrease the risk of injury. Instead of your precious energy leaking out with every step as your body desperately works to stabilize and keep you upright, the energy will propel you toward the finish.

On my first visit to Mark's Athletes' Performance Institute in Tempe, Arizona, I was asked to perform a simple balance exercise, standing on one leg. No problem, I thought, until a coach pointed out that my form was far from perfect. The staff helped me maintain the correct posture, showing me how to better engage my muscles and align my body from head to toe. I learned how to keep my back straight and hips parallel to the floor—coaching tips similar to those you'll find in this book.

It's tougher than it sounds. I assumed the proper positions, but it took so much energy and strength that, after only a few seconds, I couldn't hold them any longer. My heart rate had risen; I was starting to sweat. I realized how every time I struck the ground while running, much of my energy was being spent simply to stabilize and keep me upright. Energy was leaking everywhere.

Then I wondered: If I had gotten this far in my career as a pro athlete without the ability to stand correctly on one leg, how great could I be if I knew proper biomechanics? I set a goal of building a solid foundation that would stand up to the rigors of swimming, biking, and running that I needed to master my sport.

You'll find early on in this program, as I did, that you'll have trouble performing some of the most basic movements, such as standing straight while keeping your shoulders, hips, knees, and ankles aligned. I marveled at how I could run for miles and yet not be able to do these seemingly simple things. The problem was that I never had

trained my body to be able to do it. I had gone through the motions of swimming, biking, and running, but the link to elite-level performance is having an understanding of what goes into each movement. With this program, you'll understand movements better, and you also will be quicker to notice when something isn't right. Instead of ignoring it, you'll know what to do and fix it before it becomes a problem or leads to decreased performance.

You'll come to recognize, as I did, which muscles should be engaged during an exercise in order to maximize stability and efficiency of the movement. In just a few weeks, I was swimming, biking, and running stronger, faster, and with less effort. More important, I have been free of overuse injuries since I began the program, and I am confident that if I continue to incorporate Mark's techniques into my training, not only will I be injury-free for the rest of my career, but I will also be able to continually push the limits of my performance.

As a busy endurance athlete, you might be wondering how you're going to add this to your already busy schedule. The beauty of Core Performance is that it integrates your existing training into a total package. It might replace certain components, saving you time. What I love most about Core Performance is that I have learned to be more efficient with every workout and with every repetition. Who has time to do things that don't directly contribute to improved performance?

In the process, I've been able to cut my overall training time by about a third, yet I'm stronger and faster than ever. You will learn to accomplish more with the time you have. If you have only 45 minutes to work out, the best thing isn't necessarily to just do a 45-minute run. Performing a few "Core" exercises for the first 10 minutes will allow you to be better warmed up, standing taller and feeling fresher right from the start for a quality 30-minute run. Otherwise, you'd spend the first 10 minutes in leisurely jog mode, feeling a bit stiff and thus running with less than perfect form. That leaves 5 minutes at the end for some stretching, and here, too, the Core Performance system will show you methods that are more efficient and effective.

Not only have you had a great workout, you've decreased the potential for injury, reinforced your strengths instead of your inefficiencies, and jump-started recovery for the next workout. I begin and end each of my training sessions with 5 to 30 minutes of Core Performance exercises. No matter how little time I have, I know I will be better off doing at least something instead of rushing into my workout. I've learned to make every second count. It's not about how much you train, it's about how well you train.

The best compliment I've received since starting the Core program was from a fellow runner, who watched my pre-workout routine and asked if I had once been a dancer. My background is in competitive swimming, and before Core, I had the typical broad back, hunched shoulders, little flexibility, and no coordination.

My sister, who *is* a dancer, always stands tall, with perfect posture. She has great balance and stability and the flexibility of a contortionist. Though I was proud of my strength and swimming ability growing up, I always was in awe of her body control and physique. Now I have it all: balance, stability, power, strength, flexibility, and a killer physique that is incredibly lean and powerful. I still can't dance, but at least now I have the confidence to try.

Thanks to Mark and Core Performance, I'll never have to wonder, "What if?" I have what I need to reach my goals as an athlete and, even better, to live my best life. I know as I get older I won't still be a professional athlete, but this system has taught me that these same philosophies and training programs can help anyone, regardless of where they are in life. As much as Core Performance has helped me as a professional athlete, I'm even more excited to have this knowledge for my life beyond my athletic career.

I want to be able to hoist grandkids and my great-grandkids, even race with them. I want to be standing tall and strong the rest of my life. I want to be able to decide when, if ever, I want to stop participating in sports because my mind says I've had enough and not because my body says so. Now I know I can.

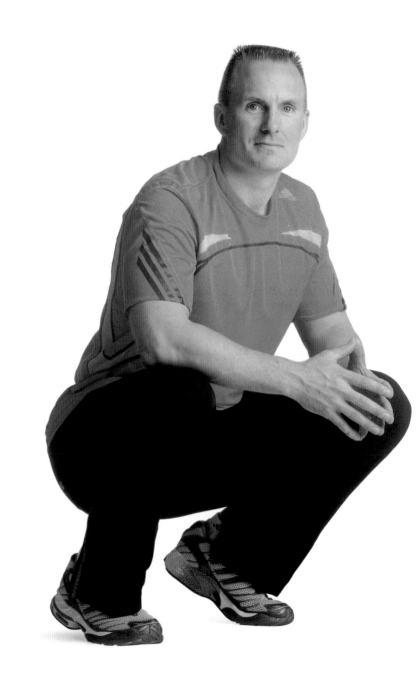

THE ENDURANCE PARADIGM SHIFT

have the utmost respect for endurance athletes. They push their bodies and minds beyond their limits, always striving for a way to run, swim, or cycle faster and farther.

If you've picked up this book, chances are you're one of these people, or you want to be one of them. I admire your dedication and quest for greatness, and I hope you'll allow me to show you how to become even better.

But it will take some effort on your part. After all, if you're anything like the world-class endurance athletes that my staff and I work with at our Athletes' Performance Institutes, then you're no doubt a little stubborn.

In this book, I'm going to ask you to change your mindset. We'll address your biomechanics, energy systems, nutrition, and everything you need to become a more efficient, enduring, force-producing champion.

First, however, I need you to discard much of what you believe and subscribe to when it comes to endurance training.

I know, I know: One of your greatest strengths is your existing mindset, this incredible desire and ability to put forth effort—to say nothing of the routines and regimens that have gotten you this far. All of that has made you successful in life and is the foundation of what has made you passionate about being an endurance athlete.

But you have to realize that your greatest strength often is also your biggest liability. You've accepted as reality parts of your sport that you don't find especially productive, let alone pleasant. For instance, many endurance athletes accept nagging injuries and ailments as the cost of greatness. No pain, no gain. The only way to improve is to fight through the pain, right?

Wrong. Take an honest assessment of your current training and physical condition. Do gains come slower, if at all, even though you're working hard? Do you suffer from chronic injuries such as shinsplints, patella tendinitis, foot and knee pain, groin tightness, or hamstring pulls? Does this discomfort radiate through your back and neck? Do your shoulders hurt every time you take a stroke in the pool?

Are you someone who suffers from a chronic sports injury as a result of the repetition and pounding? Do you endure frequent colds or long-term illnesses that come as a result of breaking down your body's immune system and willing it to levels that are unhealthy, to the point where your body responds the only way it knows how—by breaking down with injury or illness? Has this cycle of working hard, getting better, and suffering setbacks left you questioning your commitment to endurance training?

You can't keep asking your body for more of what it doesn't have. You want to run, ride, or swim faster or longer, but you keep doing the same thing and expecting different outcomes. What's the saying? That which got you here isn't what's going to get you to the next level. What you did when you first started training is not what you do today, and what you do today may need to be improved to get you where you want to be tomorrow. Remember that first rule of investing, the warning that comes at the end of any commercial for financial services: "Past performance is no guarantee of future return."

The same is true with your endurance training. Don't keep working harder with the same systems and mechanics that already have lead to one breakdown and will lead to further frustrations.

Maybe you're fortunate not to have sustained any injuries or ailments. Instead, you suffer from another malady: the inability to push beyond the plateau. Rather than soaring to new heights, you assume you've topped out and you go through the same routines week after week and year after year as a way of maintaining a base level of fitness. Thousands, perhaps millions of people, go for a daily, leisurely 3-mile run or get on a piece of exercise equipment for an hour without really breaking a sweat.

That's better than doing nothing, of course. But it's no way to improve your overall health. So if you fall into either of these categories—the chronically ailing or the athlete who is just going through the motions—I'm going to provide solutions.

Maybe you're just getting into endurance training. Or perhaps you're stepping it up a notch, from running 5-Ks to 10-Ks or sprint triathlons to Olympic distance triathlons. If so, I'm excited, because you probably haven't experienced these setbacks and ailments. Through this system, you'll learn how to avoid them.

So, how are we going to change things? Let's use the marathon as an analogy. Everyone in the race is running at the same relative intensity with the same perceived exertion level over 26.2 miles. What separates the elite runner from the recreational jogger—or the elite from the recreational in swimming or cycling—is not simply a natural gift or mental toughness as much as the mastery of an efficient system that allows the body to cover more ground and get more out of each stride or stroke.

Elite athletes have far greater pillar strength, which is to say stability and mobility through their hips, torso or "core," and shoulders. Their bodies move in perfect harmony from head to toe. That results in fewer "energy leaks" and allows them to put more force into the ground or pedal or water and propel themselves forward. It actually takes elite athletes less energy to cover the same distances faster.

Most people rationalize their lesser performances. They don't have as much time to train or haven't been involved in the sport for as long. The other person, they figure, is more genetically gifted. I'm here to tell you that you can obtain those same high-performance levels if you readjust your routines and adapt some easy-to-learn principles.

Since the publication of my first two books, *Core Performance* and *Core Performance Essentials*, I've heard from many endurance athletes. Most pose a variation of the same question: "How can I incorporate the Core training system into my crazy schedule of running/cycling/swimming, to say nothing of work, social, and family commitments?"

I'm not asking you to commit *more* time. Instead, I'll show you how to *save* time. Our goal is to complete the same amount of work in less time and get better results. This speaks to the Core Endurance workout itself and also to the systems that form the foundation for your success.

We'll do this by creating a system that includes high-performance nutrition, along with drills and activities that get your body's operating system and muscles working more effectively to reduce stress. At the heart of the philosophy is the notion of Prehab. Instead of suffering injuries and undergoing rehabilitation or rehab, we're going to be proactive in the care of our bodies to minimize the potential for injury.

In short, we want you to get more out of what you're already doing. Think about how well you take care of your automobile or bicycle. You're always taking it into the shop for preventive maintenance and upgrades. A bicycle might need a new hub or shifting mechanisms. Perhaps it requires lighter wheels or tires. But before you can consider any of that, you have to make sure you have the best frame to build from. Otherwise, you defeat the purpose of the upgrades and, in fact, could make the situation worse.

The same is true with your car. You don't think twice about paying for regular oil changes and maintenance. It's a significant cost, but you undertake it because you want the car to run optimally and for as long as possible.

Isn't it amazing that most of us, even dedicated athletes, don't make a comparable investment in our own short-term and long-term maintenance? We take better care of equipment with limited life spans than we do of our own bodies. We don't even take advantage of our powerful on-board computer—our minds—that can program the vehicles of our success—our bodies—to greater performance.

Even in a relatively short 500-mile NASCAR race, drivers have regular pit stops. Cyclists and triathletes are obsessive about bicycle maintenance. Avid runners replace shoes at the first sign of wear.

But how often do you service the ultimate vehicle that powers your riding, running, cycling, or whatever endurance sport you enjoy? Do you do it daily or weekly? Or do you just keep driving your body harder only to become frustrated or surprised when it breaks down, whether it's from nagging aches and pains or a traumatic injury that serves as a wake-up call because your body had to override your mind?

This book will give your body the same checklist you have for your bike. Just as you make sure the brake pads are intact, I want you to listen to your body and make sure all systems are running properly, so you can enjoy this wonderful world of endurance training.

You'll learn that less is more. I'm not asking you to place more demands on your time. With *Core Performance Endurance*, we will create systems and routines that will save you time over weeks, months, and years. You'll find that at the end of the year, you have achieved a higher quality of training than in years past.

We want to take a proactive approach to minimizing all those performance-hindering injuries and remove you from a system that no longer is receptive to change because it's so run-down.

Think about how much time you spend running, riding, or swimming. What if I asked you to spend 10 to 20 minutes before your workout that would cut your training time from, say, 2 hours to 90 minutes but would give you a far greater return on investment in your health and performance than spending that additional half-hour on your endurance workout? Wouldn't you jump at that opportunity?

Before you hit the road or jump in the pool, you're going to spend 10 to 20 minutes that will decrease your injury potential and improve your workout so that your body is more receptive to the upcoming training stimulus, and you'll achieve far greater results. You'll get more out of each workout, whether that translates into doing more in less time because your body is sufficiently prepared or getting far more out of the workout time you had already scheduled.

At the moment, you probably don't realize that when you take off on a run, one or both of your gluteus muscles (or "glutes") are not firing properly, and that cuts your stride length down. If your muscles are not firing properly, your body will have so many energy leaks that your effectiveness will suffer during your workout.

The *Core Performance Endurance* system provides a preflight checklist that ensures that everything is turned on and in harmony. Your system will start off operating at peak efficiency, so you can maximize the return on your upcoming exercise investment.

Let's start improving your return on that investment right now.

PART 1

THE CORE ENDURANCE MINDSET

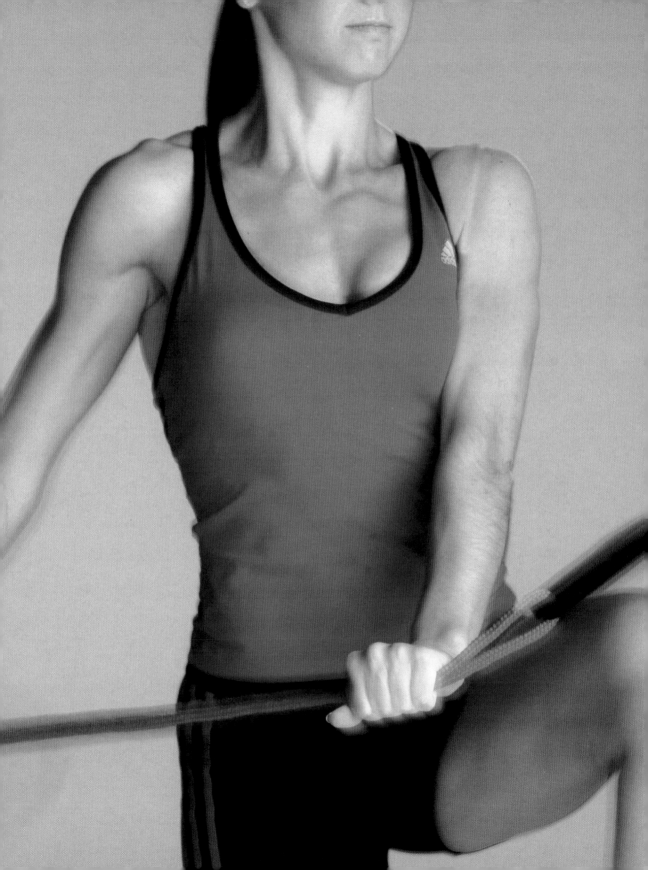

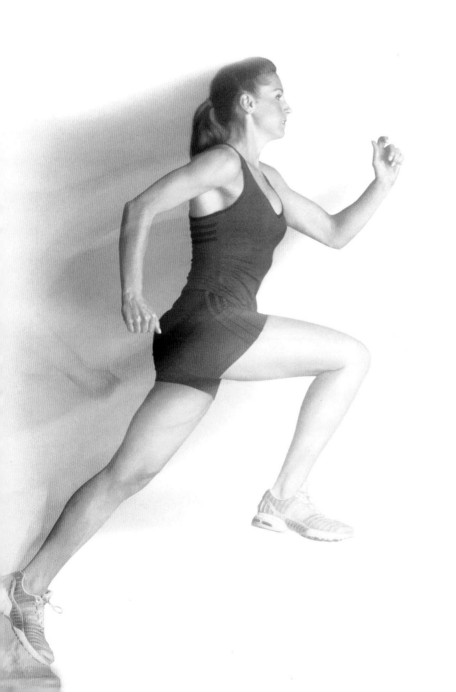

CHAPTER 1

A CALL TO CHANGE

Take your left hand and place it on a flat surface, preferably a table. Raise your middle finger and push it down as hard as you can. Really slam that finger down.

Now relax your hand. Reach over with your right hand, pull that same finger back and let it snap down. Go ahead. Do it again and again. How much effort did it take to do that? Not much, but it generated so much more force than through the first method.

If you were to keep raising that middle finger on its own, you'd get tired. But if you can store and release that energy, lifting with your other hand, you can do it all day long and produce many times the power with a fraction of the effort.

This is a good illustration of elastic power.

We want to be able to store and release energy efficiently. Everything we do has some sort of elastic component to it, whether it's walking, running, going down steps, or playing sports. The more efficiently we can store and release energy, the less effort we have to expend.

Elasticity, this ability to store and release energy efficiently, is the reason people are able to run marathons in just over 2 hours. The foundation of elasticity is stability and mobility. Go back to our finger exercise: If you lift your finger and don't stabilize your hand on the table, you'll lift your hand as well as your finger off the table. Stability allows you to have a fixed point from which to stretch the muscle, so it can efficiently store and release that energy. Stability is your foundation.

Mobility is the ability to take that finger back through the range of motion, allowing for fluid movement and greater potential to store and release energy. Mobility can be restricted because of tight tissue or poor joint mechanics, problems that could come from traumatic injury or misuse through inefficient biomechanics over time.

Once we harmonize stability and mobility, we have the foundation for elasticity. These efficient movement patterns empower you to run, ride, and swim faster with less energy expenditure. This is all part of the Holy Grail of endurance training. And we'll show you how to get there.

ELASTICITY AND TISSUE TOLERANCE

Through this program, you'll develop *tissue tolerance*. Your body breaks down when it's overstressed or under-recovered. Training creates small microtears in your tissue, and ultimately, you're going to overstress or rip the fabric unless you address this problem.

Elasticity, along with mobility and stability, decreases the tissue load. When your body is more elastic, each stroke and stride puts less of a load on your tissue. Think of your body as a pogo stick. We want our bodies to be able to store and release energy powerfully, just like a pogo stick.

When you have good elasticity, your body stretches and snaps back well. But if the tissue is tight, with a dozen knots in it, it doesn't have the ability to store energy and it does not snap back. If you took a rubber band and stretched it, you'd notice its ability to lengthen and to store energy evenly. But if you tied knots in it and tried to stretch it, it wouldn't be nearly as effective.

In this program, we're going to make sure that knots don't form. You don't want to do the equivalent of letting your tissue sit in the sun and dry out. If you do, it's going to get brittle and lose its elasticity. If you tug on it, it's going to break.

If you're not building tissue tolerance—not taking care of your muscular and connective tissue—then you're going to be limited in endurance activities. Tissue tolerance is the foundation of your body's ability to perform and protect itself from injury.

I'm guessing you haven't given a lot of thought to tissue tolerance. Take a moment and consider your relationship with your tissue. Right now, you might not have a lot of respect for it. You do some stretching, but mostly on autopilot, not making significant improvements. Perhaps you get occasional massages; sometimes, they're painful.

I want you to have a better understanding of how important tissue is to your endurance success. Think about your tissue as a carving knife. If you keep using it without cleaning it regularly and sharpening it periodically, it's going to be rendered useless before long. If you ignore your tissue like this, the neglect will translate into injury that will set you back until your body can recover. Even if you don't get injured, your performance will suffer, like a dull knife.

If you don't do proactive maintenance on a consistent basis, this is what will happen. With the Core Performance Endurance (CPE) system, you'll learn how to obtain tissue quality and stay proactive, which will have you swimming, running, and biking with less pain and fewer setbacks over the course of the year.

Your relationship with your tissue is no different than a relationship with a significant other: If you neglect it, you're going to hear about it. Muscles let you know through spasm or injury. Give your muscle tissue a little love, and you'll be rewarded with a smoother, more productive training experience—just as the proper investments of time, communication, shared feelings, and gestures nurture a relationship and prevent major confrontations.

Many athletes have abusive relationships with their bodies. They assume their bodies will always be there for them. When their bodies don't respond, they get angry and disappointed, even though the solution to this relationship trouble is right in front of them. Don't get mad at your body for an injured hip or pulled hamstring. Instead, look in the mirror and ask yourself what you have done for your muscle lately. Are you guilty of neglecting a key relationship?

You can't turn the other (butt) cheek with tissue tolerance or dysfunctional movement patterns. Just as every fractured relationship shows early signs of trouble, your body gives hints in the form of spasms and tweaks. If ignored, they're going to progress into something more serious. But if you heed the warnings and take action, you'll keep these spats from becoming all-out wars.

Tissue tolerance is the limiting factor for people trying to complete a marathon, half-marathon, or triathlon. It's not that their lungs can't handle it, or they run out of gas; it's that their muscle tissue can't withstand such a heavy volume of work. The inefficiencies and movement dysfunctions in the system cause the tissue to work harder and burn more energy. That fatigue creates more stress and requires more effort.

As a highly active person involved in endurance training, you probably don't think of yourself as lacking stability, flexibility, or tissue tolerance. After all, you're not one of the millions of overweight, inactive Americans who spend most of their time in front of televisions and computers, never getting any exercise. You've taken charge of your health. You live for competition. *Carpe diem* is your middle name.

But you still may not realize how inefficient your body has become. You're like an expensive, self-propelled lawnmower. When the lawnmower is new, it cruises through your grass. It's all you can do to hang on to the thing as it rumbles over your lawn, requiring little effort on your part.

Gradually, though, the machine loses power. It doesn't move quite as fast, and you have to push it a little bit, especially if you've neglected the routine maintenance. Over time, the mower deteriorates to the point where you're pretty much pushing a heavy piece of machinery across the lawn. Since the mower's decline is so slow and subtle, you don't realize how much power and efficiency you've lost. After all, it's a top-of-the-line mower. But it's no longer performing like one.

The same thing happens to our bodies. As babies, we learn these wonderful movement patterns. When you see young children at a park, look at their flexibility: It's amazing. Look how they're able to lunge, squat, and run. It comes naturally to them. Back when the United States was more of an agricultural and manufacturing society, people continued to use these movement patterns through adulthood in their daily labor.

Now look at what's happened: Technologi-cal advances have made it possible for adults to sit all day, whether it's at a desk and in meetings or on planes and in automobiles. Since we no longer draw upon our fundamental movements, we lose them. And even if you run, swim, or bike, you don't re-establish these movements unless you take specific action.

In fact, by engaging in endurance sports without re-establishing these movements, you put yourself at greater risk for injury and, arguably, illness than the person who never breaks a sweat.

THE SYSTEM AT THE CENTER

In the Foreword, you heard from Jessi Stensland, who, despite being an accomplished triathlete when she arrived at our Athletes' Performance Institute, could not stand on one leg. It was as if she had high-performance bicycle tires and wheels, but her spokes could not support them. Jessi, like a lot of endurance athletes, figured that the secret to getting better was to just train harder.

Endurance athletes have a martyr complex. "Yeah, my left hip is killing me, but I'm tough. I'll just battle through it; I'll be all right." That kind of mentality might work for a football player trying to slog his way through an important game, but it isn't going to work for an endurance athlete trying to maximize his or her potential.

Most runners figure that the way to get better is through more running. It's the same mentality we see today with youth sports. Parents all but force kids to specialize in one sport at an early age, figuring that the extra time spent will enable them to thrive. In reality, they're shutting down movement patterns that don't relate to their one sport. I'm amazed how often I see young, accomplished one-sport athletes who look downright uncoordinated when they attempt to play something else. Or worse—their bodies are incapable of performing the basic movements for the sport. That didn't happen 15 years ago.

Now, I'm not asking you to take up a different sport. As adults, it's all we can do to find time for *one.* But whatever sport you choose, take the time to re-establish and improve your fundamental movement patterns. Your health and performance depend on it.

If you're a recreational endurance athlete, you can improve your performance for years to come with the scientifically backed system in this book. As you work the system, you will consistently enjoy great gains, thrive in your endurance events, and improve the quality of your life.

If you're an elite endurance athlete, consider the system a means to maximize your return on investment. At this point in your career, you'll find that the return is far greater if you address the core fundamental movement patterns than if you add another 15 to 20 minutes to your workout. At this point, it's not about performing more, it's about performing *better.*

In order to optimize your performance, every aspect of your training needs to have a specific prescriptive purpose. This is how good athletes become great. All of the athletes who come to the Athletes' Performance Institutes are searching for ethical, meaningful ways to upgrade their current systems and rituals to keep them at the cutting edge of human performance. They know that if they don't improve, they will plateau and fall behind.

The reason the Core Performance Endurance system works for both recreational and elite athletes is because it's proactive. You won't allow yourself to keep going and going, accepting pain as part of your sport. You won't wait to address the pain until you've hurt your back or pulled a muscle. Instead, you'll heed the warning signs the entire way.

If you want to achieve peak performance, you have to take care of your most valuable machinery. As we discussed in the Introduction, it's time to wake up and go through a pre-workout checklist for the most important tool that you have in endurance sports and in life—your body. You'll listen to what it has to tell you, and then you'll develop the systems it needs to perform at a consistently high level. Along the way, you'll be able to avoid about 65 percent of the injuries that you're exposed to as an endurance athlete. (More on this in Chapter 4.)

Like a strong, stable hub on the wheel of a racing bike, the Core Performance Endurance system brings structure and efficiency to what once was a collection of parts. We'll align your body and your movements so that, like a wheel, you will continue to roll once you are set in motion. As with a bike hub, the system itself doesn't move much, but everything depends on it. It fine-tunes the wheel. Set the wheel in motion with the system for support, and it will roll along in perfect alignment, effortlessly eating up the miles.

When you work inside the system, you'll feel calm at the center, and you'll fly along. You will have done all the legwork necessary to get to, and stay in, "the zone." You'll move so efficiently that you'll feel like going all day long.

Longtime runners assume they know how to run. "I've been doing it a long time, thus I must have a good understanding of it." If you're one of these people, how actively have you sought to improve your biomechanics? Do you understand how the body transfers force? I want you to understand what your body is doing and how it works most efficiently. Don't just listen to hearsay. "Oh, that's just the way we do it." Too often, endurance athletes go until they drop, dealing with the pain and dysfunction. It shouldn't be that way.

The alternative to this system is pressing onward until you get hurt. Then you have to address what your body has been trying to tell you all along. It's not just about doing more volume and quantity and then tapering off and you'll be better. That philosophy does have a place, but only for someone who is already operating with maximum efficiency.

We want every stride to be perfect, and early on, this might take a tremendous amount of mental energy, just as it did the first time you embarked on a run. You've probably grown accustomed to running on autopilot, daydreaming. Instead, you need to focus and concentrate on biomechanics. This program is about becoming engaged, programming your body and upgrading the system so that you can get more out of each stride with less effort. It will be mentally exhausting, but over time, it becomes second nature. You'll build and hone these efficient movement patterns until you *become* them.

Think of it this way: Do you endurance train to work more and harder? Or is your goal to get better? If you want to improve your health, as well as your times and performance, I need you to think differently.

This mindset shouldn't be much of a stretch, since we examine every other aspect of our lives—finances, job, family, possessions—and search for ways to improve in the fastest, most efficient manner. Home improvement has become a national pastime. We understand that the route to wealth is not by working longer and harder, but by acquiring knowledge and creating assets that enable us to work more efficiently.

Have we considered our endurance training systems in a similar light? Or do we just take it for granted that we have limited genetic potential, and we'll just keep doing what we're doing? Let's discard that thinking. *Core Performance Endurance* will give you the most effective way to upgrade your training. It will take less time, it will decrease wear and tear, and you'll get more return on investment.

So let's shift the paradigm of doing more and more sloppy volume—the traditional focus of endurance training. There's no way that by tapering off you'll miraculously discover some effective technique and speed. So many endurance training magazines and Web sites focus on one element of the specific skill to improve that will produce results. What's really needed is a complementary foundation, a system that supports those skills.

THE FOUNDATION FOR ENDURANCE

Establishing a foundation for endurance success has little to do with working up a huge base of volume. Instead, your base will be the core fundamental movement skills, and a body that you've developed to be more stable, elastic, powerful, and efficient. You'll be able to translate your newfound efficiency to your endurance sport of choice.

When you neglect the foundation of your training, it's not going to be a successful undertaking. Your training will look like an inverted pyramid, with no focus on the core fundamental patterns you had as a child, when you learned to crawl, walk, jog, and run. You may presume that you've mastered these skills when, in fact, you haven't looked at the mechanics of running since you were 4 years old. Who said you had it down right then? Yet you probably moved more naturally at that age than you do today because of the constant trauma of trying to improve.

Let's go back to the beginning and re-establish your core fundamental movement patterns. That will become the basis for your long-term health and performance.

CHAPTER 1 SUMMARY: Endurance athletes typically wear themselves into the ground. Instead of trying to improve biomechanics and core fundamental movements, many follow the traditional formula of working out more and more with inefficient movement patterns until their bodies break down. In the Core Performance Endurance (CPE) system, we're going to re-establish our core fundamental movement patterns, create elasticity in our bodies, and build tissue tolerance. This will enable us to work out more efficiently and thus improve performance while making us resistant to injuries, illness, and long-term deterioration.

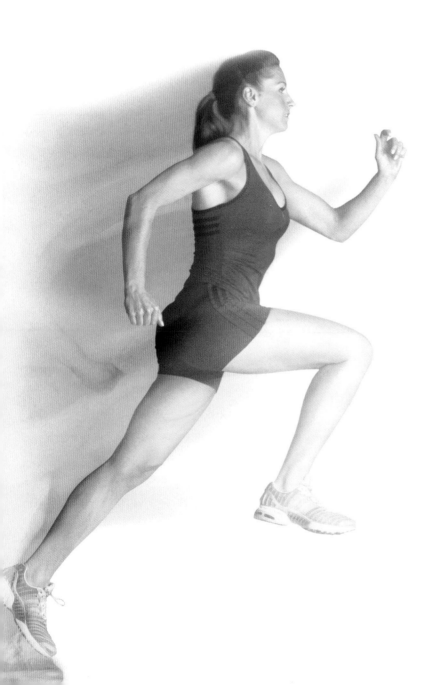

CHAPTER 2

SELF-EVALUATION

Try this test. Stand in front of a mirror, as tall as you can, with good posture. Now, lift your right leg until it forms a 90-degree angle with your hip. We call this the "triple flexion response." It's when your hip, ankle, and knee are all flexed.

Hold this pose for 60 seconds. Keep the book in your hands; don't stop reading. I want you to be able to examine your mechanics and compare them with some of the do's and don'ts we'll discuss in this chapter.

This is your basic running motion. Let's take a look at your body's alignment. Is your left hip, the leg you are standing on, in a straight line with your torso, or is it jutting out to the side? Is your left knee inside your foot? Is the foot of your "down" leg flat and rolled in to your arch, or have you created an arch in the middle?

Now let's focus on your right leg, which is in the air. What is the angle of your shin to the ground? Is it leaning in or out? Is your knee in toward the midline, or is it outside your hip? Are you starting to feel fatigue in your right or left hip yet? Is the toe of your lifted leg pointed down—or up toward the shin?

There are small muscles in your feet, knees, and hips that must stabilize every stride you take to act as the foundation. That allows muscles to efficiently store and release energy. Take a mental picture of what that looks like and the relative stress after 60 seconds of balancing on that leg. Now switch legs and repeat the process.

Did you notice a difference between your right and left sides in terms of posture, leg alignment, and the fatigue you felt in your hip? Almost every athlete I see, even world-class performers, shows imbalances, presenting a greater potential for injury. Those imbalances make you more than twice as likely to suffer an injury than if your body were in proper alignment. As you continue to run or ride and induce fatigue, the imbalance is only going to get worse. It will increase tissue load and trauma, which creates overuse injuries and decreased performance.

Did you have difficulty with that exercise? If you found that tough to maintain in a controlled setting, as most people do, imagine how inefficiently you're moving in a changing environment, when fatigue and ground surfaces are factored into the equation.

I want you to be able to hold that position on both sides with the same level of effort, which should be minimal as you master this program. If it took effort to hold balance on either side, that drains your battery. Both sides should be equally easy. You want to have *symmetry*.

During that exercise, were you able to maintain a straight line from your nose through your chest, belly button, and inseam? Most people drop a hip down to lift the leg. If you're on the left leg, the right hip drops, and the left hip juts out to the side. We call that "sitting on your tissues." You're relying on ligaments and capsular tissues for stability instead of having your muscles functioning properly to take the load off the capsule and ligaments. The muscles are capable of acting like shock absorbers and stabilizers, decreasing the wear and tear on your joints and surrounding muscle—but only when you take the time to care for them. If you were dropping your hips, you have poor hip and/or torso ("core") stability.

You also should have been able to maintain a straight line from your ankle all the way up to your armpit. Were you rocking on your heel, or were you forward on your toes? What you want to feel is an even distribution over the middle of your arch.

What was the angle of your shin in relation to your down leg? Was your knee pointing in toward the other leg, with the heel out? Or was your knee wide and your heel in toward the other leg? Our goal is to have your leg pull up in a vertical line from the floor so that it runs parallel to your down leg. You should see nothing but parallel lines when you look in the mirror. Lastly, is your foot pulled up toward your shin or is it dangling toward the ground?

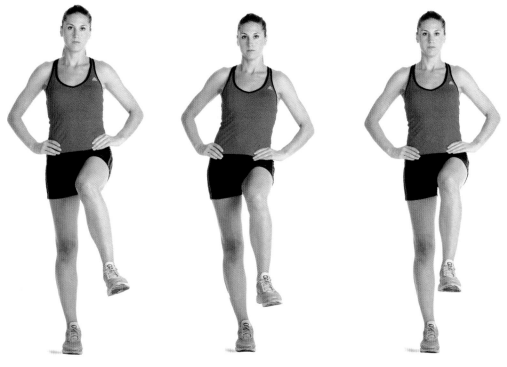

BAD   **GOOD**

This might seem nitpicky, but how your toe is positioned—up or down—goes a long way toward determining whether you'll suffer injuries. Keeping the toe up or "dorsiflexed" is arguably one the most important elements of running mechanics. It's the equivalent of a pitcher's hand interaction with the ball or a tennis player's racquet grip and subsequent serve.

Grab a partner and take this simple self-test to see how well you dorsiflex. Lie face-down on the ground and pull one leg up, as if performing a leg curl. Try to hold your leg at a 90-degree angle to the floor, as if in the middle of a leg curl, and have your partner try to pull your foot back toward the ground. Don't let your partner move it. You'll notice that your hamstring will fire, and for most people, the toe will pull up toward the shin and two big muscles will pop from the back of your calf.

Now assume the same position, your leg again at a 90-degree angle to the floor. Point your toe up toward the ceiling and have your partner hold it there. Then have your partner try to pull down on the heel. You'll be surprised to find that the tension on the hamstring is twice as much and that the calf muscle is shut off and mushy.

Why does this matter? Because your leg

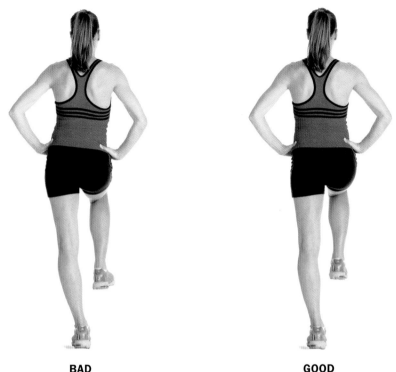

BAD   **GOOD**

goes through this action with every stride you take. If your toe is down, your calf is shut off, and your hamstring will have to do twice the work than if your calf were involved and turned on or "activated," as it is when your toe is up. With your toe down, you'll experience greater hamstring fatigue, which places an increased load on the tissue and causes slower and lower performance. You'll also be exposed to chronic hamstring tightness, which will lead to hamstring injuries.

So what does the toe's "up" position have to do with the hamstring? When your toe is pulled toward the shin, it activates your calf, specifically the gastrocnemius muscle, which crosses both your ankle and knee and acts as a secondary hamstring or leg flexor. The calf shares the load in both the recovery action and the propulsive action of your stride. This dorsiflexed position also is critical as your foot strikes the ground, allowing you to better store and release energy.

How the foot strikes the ground often confuses runners. Some try to strike with the heel. Others try to run on the toes. Neither is correct. With proper dorsiflexion, your stride's strike zone is beneath your hip, not out in front of your body. This way, you create a straight line from ear to ankle, just as you attempted during our self-test in front of the mirror.

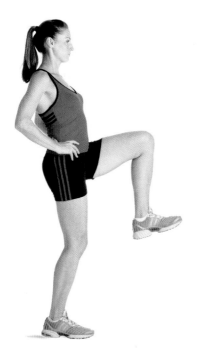

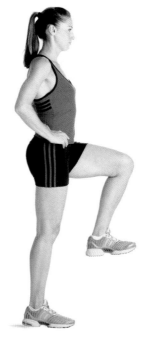

BAD   **GOOD**

Dorsiflexion allows you to stack your body's segments for extreme strength and stability. The stabilizing muscles allow force to transfer from the foot through the body out of the top of your head while minimizing the potential for energy leaks that result in tissue trauma and overuse injuries.

Dorsiflexion also applies to cycling. You produce far greater power on the downward cycle in dorsiflexed position. There is better transfer of force from the hips. As you come down into extension, you will be better able to use your glutes. With dorsiflexed position, you will be better able to use your hamstring and calf to pull up and generate greater power on the upward pulling action of the back half of your pedaling stroke. The alternative is to point your toe down in the middle or the bottom of your downward stroke, which decreases your ability to produce force, puts greater stress on the calf and hamstring, and minimizes the effect of your glutes.

So, how do we bring this dorsiflexed foot back underneath the hip? That's where we discover what I call "the benefit of the buns." Movement is all about the glutes and the power of your hips. Let's do another self-evaluation, preferably in front of a mirrored wall or at least a full-length mirror.

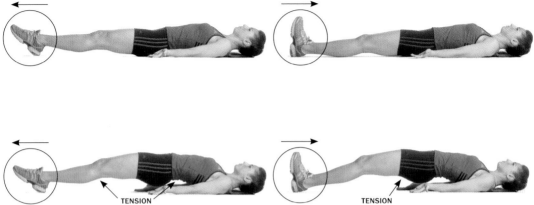

STRAIGHT-LEG BRIDGE—PLANTAR-FLEXED   **STRAIGHT-LEG BRIDGE—DORSIFLEXED**

Lie on your back, legs straight and locked out. While holding this book so you can read it, create a straight line from your ear to your ankle. Now bridge up, keeping the legs straight and lifting the hips off the ground as high as possible, continuing to read this book. Your shoulders and heels are the only two points in contact with the ground.

Do you feel the tension in your lower back and hamstrings, or are you feeling it in your glutes? Stay up now. Don't drop your hips. Set the book on your stomach. Now, take both hands and poke yourself in the glutes. See if they're both rock hard or if one is firm and the other flabby. Perhaps they're both flabby, the result of not firing (squeezing). Now relax.

Were your hamstrings and lower back going into spasm or were your glutes firing?

We're not measuring whether your rear end is fat or firm. Instead, we're trying to see whether your glutes are activated or "turned on" (hard) or not activated (soft).

Get back into the same position. Bridge up so that only your heels and shoulders are on the ground. Point your toes all the way down (as pictured in the straight-leg bridge—plantar-flexed photos above). Now pull your toes and feet up toward your shins (as pictured in the straight-leg bridge—dorsiflexed photos above). Really focus on firing your glutes. Where do you feel the tension? If your glutes are firing, you'll notice how the tension leaves your lower back and hamstrings. Relax.

Assume the same bridged position one more time. Point your feet down, and without moving your hips, lift your right leg off the

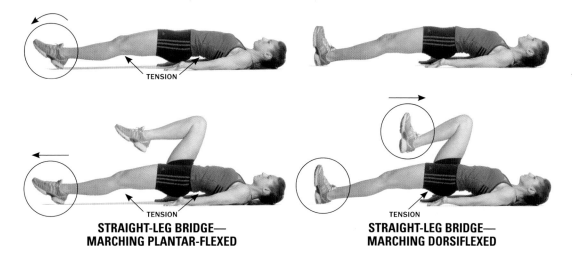

BAD

GOOD

TENSION

TENSION

TENSION

**STRAIGHT-LEG BRIDGE—
MARCHING PLANTAR-FLEXED**

**STRAIGHT-LEG BRIDGE—
MARCHING DORSIFLEXED**

ground (as pictured in the straight-leg bridge—marching plantar-flexed photos above). Switch legs and rest. I know that was difficult; you probably felt tension in your hamstrings, calves, and lower back. Yet that's the position in which most people strike the ground with their legs when they run, a position that puts undue stress on the body. Now you know why you end up with hamstring, calf, shin, and lower back problems. Your body is working too hard.

Thankfully, the solution is as simple as pulling your feet and toes toward your shins (as pictured in the straight-leg bridge—marching dorsiflexed photos above). Bridge once again off the ground, with your feet and toes pulled toward your shins. Lock out your legs by squeezing your quads. Fire your glutes, and now lift your right leg off the

ground. Now switch, driving your heel back toward the ground and really firing your glutes. Now try it again. If you had a level or broomstick on your pelvis, the idea would be to keep it level to the ground as you develop a great "rotary stability." This dorsiflexed position and firing your glutes to keep your body off the ground is the exact feeling you should experience upon foot contact with the ground. The leg, with the dorsiflexed ankle, simply acts as a lever controlled by your glute. That glute should pull the leg back under the hip and make contact with the ground, giving you more of a full-foot landing with dorsiflexion and glute activation. Your hips will propel forward as your glute fires and rolls you over the big toe, a motion we call the "triple flexion extension response" because it stretches all the muscles of the

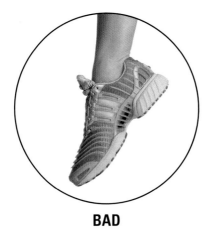

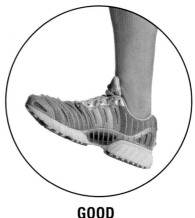

BAD   **GOOD**

lower leg. The body's three main joints—hip, knee, and ankle—create tremendous force when moved from the extended position to the flexed position. It's just like the position you held in the balance test.

Arm action ties right into this. One of the misnomers in endurance running is that you shouldn't use your arms because they will use too much energy. When you don't use your arms, you don't fully engage your muscles. Your torso and legs can't fully use this efficient storing and releasing of elastic energy that is critical to taking your performance to the next level.

Granted, we need economy of movement to thrive as endurance athletes, but don't be so short-sighted that you squander a valuable opportunity for efficient movement. By using your arms and shoulders effectively, you actually create and recycle more energy. You do this by relaxing the shoulders and

keeping your arms bent between 70 and 100 degrees, as if your hands were constantly going through your pockets. With your elbows driving back and forth along your torso, your chest and the front of your shoulders and torso can stretch. Your elbows naturally will snap back to the front of your body, creating an efficient, pendulum-like motion.

What does this all have to do with running faster? In a word: everything. Human movement is completely integrated; you'll find that your arm action dictates your leg action.

Let's do another self-test. Stand up, as if you were striding, pushing off your left leg and placing your right foot up on a chair. Now position your arms as they'd be while running, with your right elbow back and your left elbow forward. As you bring the right elbow back, note the stretch in your chest and a

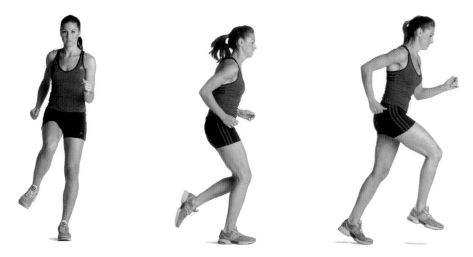

RUNNING: BAD RECOVERY AND FORM

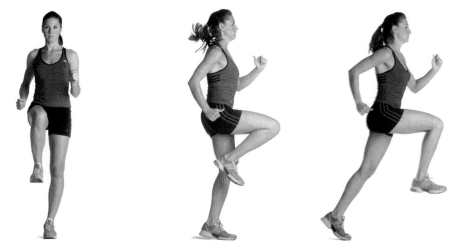

RUNNING: GOOD RECOVERY AND FORM

more modest stretch in the abdominal region. If the left glute fired, you also should feel a stretch of the left hip flexor down through your quad. Imagine a rubber band attached from your right shoulder, across your chest and abs, down around your left hip flexor and attaching below the knee.

That rubber band would be under an incredible amount of stretch. When it snaps back, the stored energy releases and pulls you into triple flexion. Now switch feet and put the other one up on the chair. Take the

SHIN PAIN

Two common types of shinsplints can be a result of poor running technique. If you have shin pain on the inside of your lower leg, you are probably a toe runner.

Pain on the outside of your lower leg means you probably have a tendency toward a hard or excessive heel strike when you run. Landing on your heel puts a large eccentric (negative) stress on the muscle responsible for slowing down your foot, resulting in an inflamed state.

You can remedy both types of pain by trying to contact the ground with the full length of your foot, with the load coming through the middle of your arch. This will help reduce the stress on the muscle that is irritated.

same action and envision that rubber band going from behind the left knee, around the back of the hamstring, across the left glute, across the lower back, over the shoulder blade and attaching to your right elbow.

The band is now quite stretched. When it snaps back, it will fire your elbow, glute, and hamstring back until that leg strikes underneath the left hip. As you fire your glute and push off your big toe into triple extension, it triggers the triple flexion response again. This is the epitome of efficient human motion, and it demonstrates how what I call your "pillar strength" (more on that in a moment) acts as the foundation of all movement. The spokes attached to this hub of your body, known as the pillar, should be used to put muscles on "stretch" from your upper body across to the lower

part of your body. This enables it to efficiently store and release energy, so you can run faster, expending less energy for longer periods.

Maybe you don't run. You're a cyclist. This applies to you as well. It's the same action you use when you attack, sprint, or climb with maximum output. You grip the bars and transfer force by pulling with the right arm and pushing with the left leg. Then you repeat the process on the other side. The energy transfers from the left handlebar to the right pedal and vice versa. That's why you pay top dollar for a frame that's rigid and has good tortional rigidity—it absorbs shock and road vibrations—so you can efficiently transfer the force into the crank and ultimately into the wheel.

This also applies to swimming. A stable pillar and shoulders offset each other to create rotation. As you pull through the water, your hips and shoulders go in opposite directions, creating another stretch across your body. Poor swimmers use only their arms. Good swimmers use their arms and legs. Great swimmers employ their shoulders, torso, and hips—their pillar—to power their arms and legs. The butterfly stroke is the epitome of an elastic expression as the body arches out of the water and puts the anterior chain—the muscles of the front of the body—on stretch. Everything wants to snap back and pull back into flexion, causing the muscles to want to snap back and repeat the process.

I'm guessing you haven't given a lot of thought to how your body moves, or to how it's supposed to move, anyway. You probably feel like you could have done better on the self-tests, and that's okay. Get excited. If you can make these simple corrections and combine that with your dedication to your endurance sport, think how much better you're going to become.

CHAPTER 2 SUMMARY: Even some of the most accomplished, gifted athletes lack mobility, stability, and some of the core fundamental movement patterns to thrive in their sports. Through some basic self-evaluations, it's possible to recognize these specific limitations and create a system that will allow the body to operate with maximum efficiency. The key is to recognize that human movement is integrated and that your pillar transfers the energy from your upper body to your lower body, creating efficient movements.

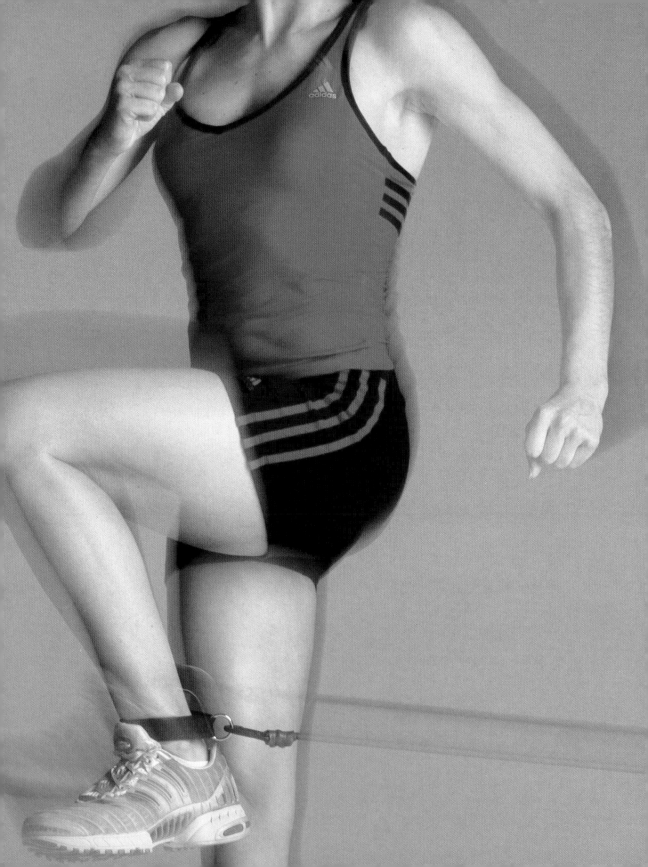

PART 2

CORE ENDURANCE MOVEMENT

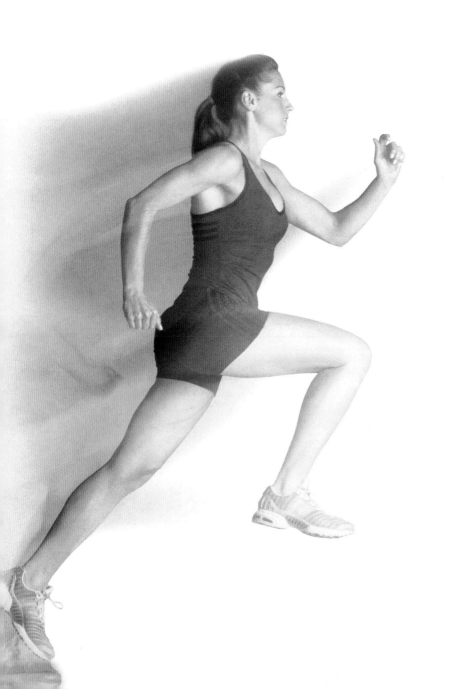

CHAPTER 3

BUILDING YOUR PILLAR

I f you've ever participated in or watched a 10-K or marathon in your local community, you've noticed that most everyone goes through the same prerace static stretching routine. They place one calf over the other, bend down, and hold the position for 15 seconds. Or they grab a foot and pull it back to their butt. Some push against a tree or wall. These familiar routines are what we were taught in junior high gym class.

These runners are about to embark on activity that requires dynamic, fluid action, and they are preparing in the most inefficient way possible. Static stretching before a workout is not the way to gain flexibility, nor should flexibility be viewed as the end-all prerace strategy.

When I watch these static stretching routines, I see people trying to commandeer their muscles and turn off the circuit breakers right before they need them most. Instead of improving race performance, they're actually making the upcoming demands harder on the body.

Think about it. These people are taking the muscles and putting them in submissive holds to the point where they shut off. The last thing we want to do prior to going out and running or riding is to discourage and shut down our muscles.

Don't get me wrong; I'm a fan of static stretching as long as it's done *after* a workout or on a lighter "regeneration" day. After all, a warm rubber band stretches farther and stores more energy than a cold one, right? But we're going to replace traditional pre-workout stretching with what I call Movement Preparation, which is an active series of warmup exercises that will efficiently increase your core temperature; lengthen, strengthen, stabilize, and balance your muscles; and, as the name suggests, prepare your body for the upcoming movement.

Movement Prep will not only improve your current workout, it will also serve as the foundation to long-term tissue quality. It will give you mastery of the core fundamental movement patterns that we all learned as children but lost as adults through inactivity and sitting in front of screens, in cars, and on airplanes. Movement Prep will ensure that your muscles are turned on and engaged, so they can deal with the demands of the upcoming workout or competition.

Movement Prep might be the most powerful tool you can use to decrease injury and improve performance. It will improve balance and proprioception, the system of pressure sensors in the joints, muscles, and tendons from which your body gathers information to maintain balance. It prepares your body for

movement by fine-tuning its nerves and feedback mechanisms. It gives you the flexibility and movement patterns for running, riding, and swimming.

Movement Prep is so powerful because it acts as the software that boots up your computer. The better this operating system works, the more you're going to get out of your body in the upcoming competition or training session. Consider this the all-important preflight checklist, a consistent way to make sure your body is optimally prepared for the upcoming demands.

Through this process, you'll also create symmetry between your right and left sides, your front and back, and the upper and lower portions of your body. This is one of the primary keys to staying healthy, decreasing the potential for injury, and moving with greater efficiency.

You'll lengthen and strengthen muscles with perfect posture and decrease injury potential by improving tissue quality. You'll see more flexibility, mobility, stability, balance, and symmetry gains by doing Movement Prep for 5 to 10 minutes a day than you've seen over years with your current warmup program.

Now do the math. Spending just 10 minutes a day, five to six days a week, over 48 weeks of the year is an investment of just 48 hours per year that will produce huge benefits in performance. Again, the goal is not to work out longer but more efficiently. Plug this into your existing routine, and you'll enjoy more benefits in less time.

Movement Prep provides the immediate short-term benefit of making you feel more fluid. You will be more prepared to stabilize every stride and increase stride length. It's the one element of this program that, if you're pressed for time and can do nothing else that day, you should never go without.

PREHAB

Through Prehabilitation, or "Prehab," you'll take action on a daily basis to decrease the potential for running, riding, and swimming injuries that could ultimately land you in rehab.

Prehab will consist of a few exercises for the critical muscles of your pillar: shoulders, torso, and hips. Prehab also will be an underlying theme in your entire endurance system. And it's more than just a series of exercises. You'll learn to think proactively about the entire Core Performance Endurance plan, from your mindset and planning to your nutrition and biomechanics to the power and strength units you'll learn shortly.

One of the central tenets of the Core Performance system is the notion of *pillar strength.* Bodybuilding-based workouts view the physique as a series of parts, and most people tend to think of movement as start-ing from the limbs. If we reach out to grab something, or we step forward, we think of those motions as originating with the end result—we've reached out, therefore, we've used our arms.

But movement starts from the very center of the body, the core area of the torso. That's why we refer to the torso as the *pillar*—its alignment and function directly correspond to the quality and efficiency of every movement. Everything is interrelated.

Pillar strength is the foundation of all movement. It consists of hip, torso (or core), and shoulder stability. (Think of a mannequin with no limbs.) Those three areas give us a center axis from which to move. If you think of the body as a wheel, the pillar is the hub, and the limbs are spokes.

We want the hub to be perfectly aligned and stable, so we can draw energy from it and effectively transfer energy throughout the body. It's impossible to move the limbs efficiently and forcefully if they're not attached to and controlled by something solid and stable.

There's a reason why parents are forever telling kids to sit up straight. Without what I call "perfect posture," which is to say this pillar strength, you will significantly increase the potential for injury in a chain of pain that starts with your lower back, descends all the way to the knees and ankles, and rises up to your shoulders, neck, and elbows.

The reason we train body *movements* instead of parts is because everything about the body's engineering is connected. What happens to the big toe affects the knees, the hips, and ultimately the shoulders. Many workout programs do more damage than good by producing muscle imbalances and inefficient movement patterns that sabotage the highly coordinated operating system with which we're born.

Everything we do in this system, especially when it comes to Prehab, will address the vital core areas of the hips, torso, and shoulders.

HIP STABILITY

The hip joints are as critical to an endurance athlete's success as the rotator cuff is to a baseball pitcher's success. That's why we call the hip joint and surrounding musculature the "hip cuff." It provides the hip with the stability, mobility, and strength necessary to act as a foundation for movement above and below the hips.

By maximizing the efficiency in and around the hip cuff through improved mobility, stability, and strength, you will discover the engine that will propel every stride and stroke of your endurance endeavors.

Your hips and glute muscles are the most important part of this powerful engine. Your "glutes" are not just there for show; they're built to go. Learning how to use the glutes

and all the surrounding musculature in the hip cuff will be one of the best things you can do to decrease injury potential and improve performance.

We want to initiate all movement from the hips, while maintaining perfect posture. If you're going up steps, squatting to pick something up, or simply walking, squeeze your glutes until your legs are extended. Walk with your toes pointed forward, your chest over your knee, and push through your hips until your leg is extended, creating a straight line from ear to ankle. This way, the pressure is on your hips—where nature intended—not the knees.

The benefit of initiating movement with your hips doesn't stop there. You know the easiest way to get buns of steel? Use them constantly. Look for every opportunity to lengthen and strengthen those glutes, whether it's squatting, hiking up hills or stairs, getting out of a chair, walking, or running. Think of life as one big glute workout, and you'll see amazing results.

Remember: It's all about the power of the glutes.

The reason we see so many running-related injuries is because people don't have the necessary hip mobility, stability, and control. Runners have to be able to effectively balance on a single leg and move from the hips. If the hips don't stabilize, the force created by the pounding of running is stored in the body. That energy is absorbed and stored in the muscles, tendons, and joints, increasing tissue load and leading to frustrating overuse injuries.

Strong glutes are vital for cyclists as well. If your glutes are weak, you're more likely to have wobbly knees while pedaling. Stable hips mean better knee alignment, which allows you to transfer more force and produce a stronger pedal stroke.

A properly functioning pair of hip capsules is the most powerful component of your body, but it's the most destructive if it's locked down. If your hip capsule is locked down, lacking mobility, it's as if a bone is welded to your pelvis—like having a cast on your hip. To get anything to move, you will use excessive motion in your back and knees.

Don't be surprised to find that some of these small muscles around the hips and glutes have been switched off. You might find the left or right glute is not firing, and you're not alone. Every world-class competitor who comes into one of our Athletes' Performance Institutes has some of these muscles shut off and/or locked down. Rest assured—we will identify and work this area in almost every aspect of your program.

CORE STABILITY

You've no doubt heard the term *core stability*. Unfortunately, the phrase has been mis-appropriated to refer to washboard abs. The abs are just a small component of the middle third of your pillar known as the core. The core consists of the muscles of the abdominals, torso, and lower back. It's the vital link between hip and shoulder stability, and it includes such muscle groups as the rectus abdominis, transverse abdominis, internal and external obliques, the erector spinae, and many small stabilizer muscles between the vertebrae of the spine.

These are the tiny muscles that often get shut off because of a back injury and never become reactivated, causing long-term back problems. These small stabilizer muscles cannot function alone; you have to help them by training your core muscles to become strong and stable, with the right types of recruitment patterns that will enable them to work in tandem with your shoulders and hips.

Instead of just focusing on the abs, we want to create the framework for all movement. The aim isn't just a well-sculpted midsection; it's a high-performance core.

Your core area is the catalyst to higher levels of performance and reduced potential for injury. It will propel you toward more fluid, efficient movement in every run, ride, or swim.

In order to maximize the benefit of the exercises in the Core Performance Endurance program, it's important to keep your tummy tight, not just while exercising, but all day. Think of your tummy flat against the hipbones. Keep your tummy tight by "feeling tall" and slightly pulling your belly button off your belt buckle. This isn't the same as sucking in your gut and holding your breath. Keep the abdominals in, but not in so far that you can't breathe.

Your abdominal and lower back muscles work as a team. The ringleader is the transverse abdominis, or "TA," which is the first muscle that's recruited each time you move. If you can keep your TA activated and your tummy tight, you'll be well on your way to efficient movement and preventing long-term deterioration.

SHOULDER STABILITY

The shoulders take a beating in endurance sports, whether you run, ride, or swim. Take a look at your posture in the mirror. Perhaps your chin is sticking forward. Your shoulders might be rolled in, with your thumbs rotated toward the center of your body.

You can end up in this position through the swim stroke, which causes internal rotation, or through a bike position in which you're hunched over the handlebars. If you're running like many people do, using your arms not nearly as much as you should, you're probably tight around the chest.

All of these forces are pushing us forward, down, and in toward the midline of the body, giving us that hunched-over look. The stresses of everyday life also contribute, whether it's sitting in front of computers or in planes, trains, and automobiles.

If you rush from the office for your workout without activating the muscles that reset the shoulder joint into proper alignment, you'll start to swim, ride, or run with your shoulders rolled in. Before you know it, you've got to work through this shoulder pain during the workout and afterward because the pain you have in the front of the shoulder won't go away.

We tend to think of the hands and arms as carrying the workload for the upper body, but it's really the shoulder, or at least it should be. That's why we often speak of someone *shouldering* a burden.

Our natural instinct is to drop the shoulders forward, especially after long periods of sitting. But you ought to do the opposite, elevating the sternum up and letting your shoulder blades hang back and down, which will give you proper posture.

As people age, they tend to flex forward, as if the chest is caving in. We ought to do the opposite, almost as if there's a fishhook inserted under the sternum, pulling us up. This will allow the shoulders to fall into place and help give perfect posture.

The exercises in this program will require you to bring the shoulders back and down,

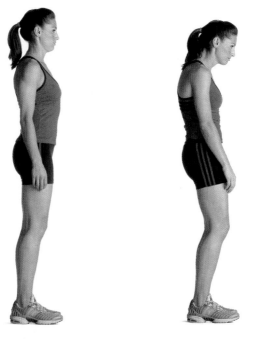

GOOD AND BAD POSTURE

but you'll want to make it a daily habit. To make lasting change, we want to lengthen the chest and strengthen the muscles of the upper back, rotator cuff, and the rest of the shoulders.

This posture is the exact opposite of the shoulder shrug, the motion you make when you say, "I don't know." That's what a sitting lifestyle does to you. If you make a habit of bringing your shoulders down—think of dropping your shoulder blades into your back pockets—you'll be amazed at the results.

We'll focus a few minutes each day on improving your shoulder, torso, and hip strength and stability. Not only will that create the foundation for power, it will also make you more resistant to injury and long-term deterioration. In these few minutes, we're investing in our health by addressing the small, stabilizing muscles in these vulnerable areas that break down in endurance sports. If we do that, we'll never have to go through agonizing rehab for foot, knee, lower back, hip, or shoulder pain.

We'll keep these exercises simple and integrate them into *fundamental* movement patterns—those basic everyday motions we had as children but that we've lost due to age and, more likely, inactivity. This Prehab process will activate specific muscle groups critical to health and performance. The prehab routines engage the muscles that sometimes get shut off due to injury or your endurance training techniques. Fortunately, it only takes a few minutes to switch these areas on for maximum power to every part of your body.

Prehab will ensure that you have a full team of muscles working together to accomplish the common goal of efficient movement. The alternative is to ignore these issues and apply the high-volume stress that endurance training requires, just waiting for the inevitable breakdown. Your body is all about teamwork, and when some muscles aren't activated, it places undue stress on other areas. That creates greater fatigue, spasms, and dysfunction in what should be

RUNNING POSTURE
By Darcy Norman

Next time you go out for a run, practice running with purpose and with more stability by focusing on these two concepts.

1. RUN TALL. Lengthen your spine by focusing on keeping the top of your head as far away from your tailbone as possible without tilting your head back. You should feel your abdominal muscles engage as you lengthen your spine.

2. PICK UP YOUR FEET. Instead of shuffling down the road, concentrate on purposefully sliding your feet toward your butt as they leave the ground and then purposefully putting them back on the ground. Initially, this will take more energy and focus, so start with this progression during your long runs.

Week 1: 1 minute of running with purpose, 4 minutes normal; repeat for length of run

Week 2: 1½ minutes of running with purpose, 3½ minutes normal; repeat for length of run

Week 3: 2 minutes of running with purpose, 3 minutes normal; repeat for length of run

Week 4: 2½ minutes of running with purpose, 2½ minutes normal; repeat for length of run

Week 5: 3 minutes of running with purpose, 2 minutes normal; repeat for length of run

Week 6: 3½ minutes running with purpose, 1½ minutes normal; repeat for length of run

Week 7: 4 minutes running with purpose, 1 minute normal; repeat for length of run

Week 8: 4½ minutes running with purpose, 30 seconds normal; repeat for length of run

Week 9+: Add 30 seconds of purposeful running each week while keeping 30 seconds of normal intervals; repeat for length of run.

Darcy Norman is a performance physical therapist.

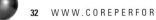

a balanced system. With Prehab, we nip those problems in the bud.

Wherever life takes you, Prehab is something you can do in a few minutes each day to maintain your body. These exercises protect you from shoulder pain, lower back trouble, hip pain, and knee and foot ailments. They will give you the necessary balance, coordination, strength, and endurance to function in everyday life and in your sport.

Prehab, along with Movement Prep, will give you the basic requirements for all human movement, the absolute minimum to sustain quality of life and performance.

CHAPTER 3 SUMMARY: Instead of traditional pre-workout static stretching, the Core Performance Endurance system uses a "Movement Prep" routine that actively and more effectively prepares the body for the rigors of the upcoming session. Pillar strength, the foundation of movement, consists of core, hip, and shoulder stability and strength. By strengthening and stabilizing these areas through a process called Prehab, we ensure that our bodies are capable of functional movement and are resistant to injury and long-term damage.

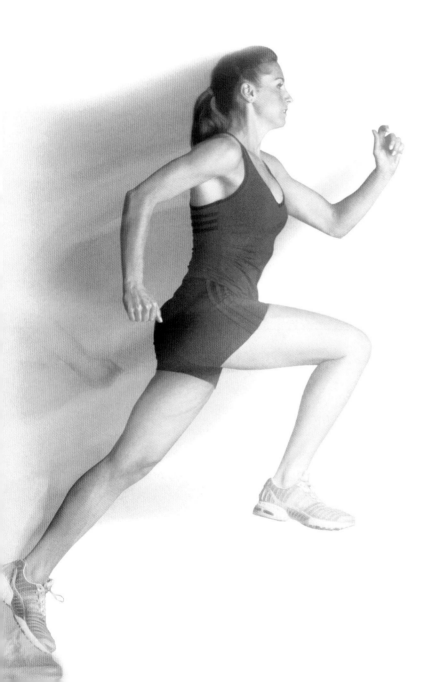

CHAPTER 4

POWER ENDURANCE

t might seem strange to see the word *power* in an endurance book. I find it stranger still that power hasn't been a focus of endurance training until recently, as endurance athletes finally are starting to respect and understand the power of wattage best measured and used in cycling. Many leading experts believe that peak and average "wattage" at efficiency ratings, like heart rate, might be the determining factor of success at the elite level.

Power is the culmination of most of your motor abilities. It's the ability to produce force efficiently. Power generated properly requires little effort on your part, enabling you to produce and transfer force into the ground or into water or a pedal all day long.

One of the things we see frequently at our Athletes' Performance Institutes are underpowered endurance athletes. Because they lack power, their bodies are forced to work much closer to their muscular and anaerobic thresholds. These athletes work so hard for every step and every climb that it takes extra effort to keep the body in motion.

Power is not a reflection of muscle size. It's about the efficiency of your nervous system to coordinate the recruitment of muscles, and about the teamwork between

RUNNING CADENCE
By Darcy Norman

Cycling studies have shown that higher revolutions per minute (RPMs) are more efficient once you have trained your body to manage that pace. The same holds true for running. For efficient running, try to make about 182 total foot contacts per minute, or 91 RPMs, regardless of your running pace. Besides making you efficient in your cadence, this will help force you to have a more efficient running form.

Darcy Norman is a performance physical therapist.

muscles to create specific and efficient movements. It's this increased coordination that allows you to be a more efficient athlete during periods of normal effort, and when you need to attack or to call upon reserves at the end of the race.

One of the key components of power is elasticity, which we discussed briefly in Chapter 1. Think of elasticity as stretching a rubber band: You store the energy in the stretch and then release it.

Our bodies work the same way, or at least they should. As you extend your body, you stretch the elastic properties of the opposite movement, and that snaps you right back to your original position. With elasticity, your body can capture energy and reuse it again and again to give you greater speed and endurance with far less energy expenditure. Think of it as recycling energy and effort.

If you don't have power and elasticity, your body will resort to the inefficient system of concentrically contracting your muscles, which is to say consciously lifting and pushing, through each stride and stroke. That takes much more energy and is significantly slower, less powerful, and less efficient.

Yet this inefficient movement represents much of what I see in endurance athletes today. We have become so focused on doing only the endurance activity, that our bodies have lost the ability to efficiently store and release energy, resulting in vehicles that don't have enough horsepower.

Without power, you don't propel your body with each stride. The goal is to propel your body from point A to point B as rapidly as possible, working with the constraints of the energy system. That's tough to accomplish with insufficient power.

As athletes who want the best from our bodies, we don't want to just lift our legs up and down repeatedly and endure. Power helps us get the most out of each stride by improving stride length and minimizing effort. A small improvement in each stride adds up quickly. The longer you run, the less energy you expend and the greater distance you can cover in the same number of strides.

It's the ultimate win-win situation. Not only that, but the higher the quality of that stride in the distance covered, the faster the recovery process will be.

Endurance training is all about *recycling* energy, or at least it should be. The elastic energy you put forth will come back to you if you can create perpetual efficient motion. Even when the body produces waste products in the form of lactate and hydrogen ions, we'll recycle it into fuel that will give us more energy. If we can continually reuse energy, we'll be optimally efficient in everything we do.

Pillar strength is vital if we are to produce power. With pillar strength, we decrease energy leaks, the areas of instability that let valuable energy trickle out, so we can't store, release, and recycle it. When energy leaks, we put more stress on other muscles, tissues, and joints. With few or no leaks, we can better transfer force, increasing energy into the ground or pedal.

Pillar strength stabilizes the body. Think of a rubber band: If you want to stretch it, you have to hold one end in place. Your muscles will do the same thing—if you have this stabilizing pillar strength. It improves your elasticity and makes you able to store and release this energy efficiently.

The stability we get from pillar strength allows us to train and compete with less energy expenditure and greater biomechanical efficiency. This in turn increases tissue tolerance, because force is distributed evenly across your body and away from the connective tissue.

The idea is to avoid riding bone on bone or "hanging on your tissues." I see that a lot with runners. Their muscles aren't firing, are too tight, or are just instable. As a result, their hip capsules must endure a ton of abuse. With each step, their femurs pound away on the pelvis like a jackhammer. That causes the joint to deteriorate, leading to pain, arthritis, and even hip replacements later in life.

There's a tendency to blame the pounding of the sport for this, but really it's the runner's fault for not maintaining the "vehicle" in optimum condition.

If we can improve the process of transferring force by minimizing energy leaks, we can decrease the potential for injury in running, biking, and swimming by upward of 65 percent. We'll be better able to reach our potential by transferring energy efficiently from the upper to the lower body, whether we're running, cycling, or swimming. The secret is a stable pillar—one that's strong through the hips, shoulders, and core.

THE ROLE OF STRENGTH

As with power, you might be surprised to find strength mentioned so prominently in an endurance book. But that's the nature of the

Core Performance Endurance system—it reconsiders much of the conventional wisdom about endurance training.

It's a mistake to think that getting strong means building huge, showy muscles. The goal of this program is to maximize your strength without gaining unwanted mass. Strength does not mean size! We are going to improve your *functional* strength, which is a combination of stabilizing strength and propulsive strength. This functional strength will give you a strong foundation for both power and endurance.

Consider functional strength a safety buffer. Your functional strength will act as a foundation for these basic movement patterns, whether they're power- or elasticity-related or part of your sport-specific training.

We also want to build *relative* strength. We're not looking to see how powerful we can become, with no regard to weight. After all, additional weight won't help with endurance sports. Instead, we want to see how powerful we can become *per pound* of body weight. That's the most important ratio. The stronger the muscle, the more it can withstand without breaking down.

Think of your body as a bicycle frame. The best titanium or carbon fiber frames are very light, but they're also very strong, with great torsional stability. They can withstand the shocks and vibrations from the road. That allows every component that's added to the bike, including the rider, to perform better. A heavier frame, with similar properties, is less efficient. The weight-to-strength ratio is not nearly as advantageous.

We want our bodies to be the equivalent of these lightweight yet powerful bicycle frames. Such a human "frame" will decrease injury potential and improve performance. Your relative strength and power will be tremendous.

Competitive cyclists think nothing of spending an extra $1,000 on a bicycle that's 10 to 16 ounces lighter than a less expensive model. If they can get the same torsional rigidity, it's money well spent. The time you spend building this relative strength will be an equally sound investment.

So how do we build strength without gaining size? We do it by improving coordination both within a muscle and among all the muscles that perform the desired movement patterns. Our strength training routine will create both stabilizing and propulsive strength.

There's a tremendous amount of synergy within the movements in the Core Performance Endurance system, and the strength unit is an important part of it. The strength exercises in this book will help improve your stability, mobility, balance, and proprioception (the information sensors in your joints and muscles), as well as your ability to hold pillar strength through various movement patterns.

Let's step back for a minute and take a look at the whole program thus far. We want to be able to increase the range of motion and stability with Movement Prep, protect our bodies from injury with a short Prehab routine, then develop force through a strength exercise, and finally contract powerfully through the new range of motion to enhance elastic properties. This process will improve your functional range of motion, increasing flexibility and giving you the perfect blend of strength to stabilize and propel you through the entire range of motion.

Strength for Stability

Sometimes, being flexible does not improve performance or decrease injury potential. Sometimes, being too flexible leads to injury because stability and strength are missing.

Imagine that you are only strong through half of your range of motion. Because you have instability or tightness, the other half of the range of motion is extremely weak. The difference between muscle length (flexibility) and strength through that particular range is a large part of your injury potential.

If you have strength and stability through a complete range of motion, along with efficient movement patterns and the right biomechanics, you will have a low potential for

injury. If you have great flexibility, but strength through a limited range of motion, with inefficient movement patterns, that remaining range of motion gives you a larger window for injury.

A lot of the movements in this program are multijoint and require stabilizing strength. *Stabilizing strength* comes from the small musculature that supports the various joints in your body, as well as the larger muscles, so they work together to create a foundation for movement.

This stability is the key to success in both

the core fundamental movement patterns and sport-specific skills.

Some of the movements that we'll use to improve the stabilizing strength of your muscles may be very isolative in nature. There are times when we isolate muscles and specific movements so that we can turn on, or activate, the muscles and integrate them back into the core fundamental movement patterns. This reintegration process discourages your body from making the kind of small muscle compensations that can eventually lead to injury. Your body has great potential to accomplish goals even if it means letting some muscles do more work while others take a day off. It's like cheating and stealing to get what you need. You'll ultimately get caught—in the form of injury or a plateau in performance.

Our goal is not just to have all the muscles on board but also to make sure they're rowing in the same direction, making all those around them better. This is the epitome of teamwork; we strive to improve efficiency and performance within our bodies.

Strength for Propulsion

Propulsive strength will improve the coordination within your muscle and between your muscles, so you can generate force more efficiently. The movements within this pro-

gram involve a lot of different joints and often work across different planes of motion. Even exercises that seem to work in one plane will challenge your body to stabilize in all planes of motion so that you can better deliver force in the appropriate direction when you run, ride, or swim.

You'll notice that many of the exercises will facilitate muscle recruitment from one side of your body to the other—for instance, from the right side of your upper body, across the pillar, and down across the left side of your lower body. This will help improve your rotary stability, as well as reinforce the cross-crawl movement patterns you use in all your endurance events.

We can also divide the body up into what we call the anterior (front) part and the posterior (back) part. This is part of the kinetic chain—the process through which your body works across all the different joints, using all the muscles to create efficient movement. Some of the exercises in this program will involve pulling for the posterior chain and pushing/squatting for the anterior chain, as well as rotational movements, which incorporate and link both together in a powerful combination.

As you go through the strength workouts, you're going to feel a new challenge. Just remember to stay stable, feel tall through your torso, and as you see little movement in these stabilized body parts, realize how much activity is truly going on to hold that stability and allow your propulsive muscles to generate force. All this attention to detail will enhance the core fundamental movements you were born with, as well as the specific skills you want to develop as an endurance athlete.

CHAPTER 4 SUMMARY: Though endurance training is not commonly associated with power and strength, both are vital to successful performance. Instead of viewing strength as a function of muscle size, look at it in terms of relative strength, the pound-for-pound ability to propel your body forward faster and more powerfully.

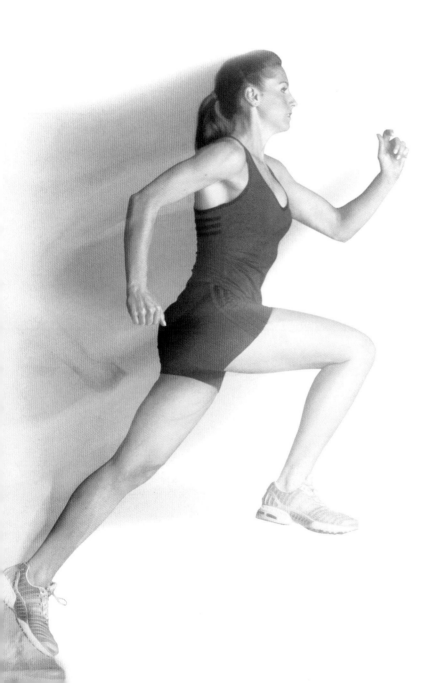

CHAPTER 5

ENERGY SYSTEM DEVELOPMENT

I dislike the term *cardio* because it's come to mean a slow, plodding workout. Think of someone who goes out for a leisurely jog or who spends a half-hour on a piece of exercise equipment while hardly breaking a sweat. People think of cardio as a way to burn calories, not to develop their energy systems.

I prefer the term *energy system development,* or ESD. As an endurance athlete, you know there's a lot more to training than so-called cardio work. In endurance sports, it's critical to realize that as we go out to run, cycle, or swim, we're not just taxing our cardiovascular systems—we're also developing motor memory, tissue tolerance, and biomechanics.

We know there are different energy systems, such as anaerobic (without oxygen), which includes *alactate* power, a short but efficient system of producing energy in increments of 1 to 15 seconds. There are different parts of the anaeroboic system that you will use based on the length of each drill. The other system we will reference is *aerobic* (with oxygen). The changeover from these systems is known as the *anaerobic* or *lactate threshold*.

The drills we'll use that will employ the alactate system will take place on our "power" days. We'll pass through this system as we work the longer lactate capacity workouts. These will be higher-intensity drills that will require maximum effort, such as sprinting, attacking, speed, power, and interval type work. You'll have to pass through this alactate segment before you can go on to the aerobic highway.

Our longest energy system, the system that people are most familiar with, is the highly efficient aerobic system. Think of the aerobic system as a reliable four-cylinder Honda Accord or Toyota Camry. Those vehicles get great mileage and perform well once they get up to speed, but they're all about long and steady performance, as opposed to furious bursts of speed during attacks or sprints. During the ESD portion of this program, you'll come to view the aerobic system as the base from which you'll accelerate to higher levels.

Our bodies combine oxygen with stored energy in the form of carbohydrates and fat to produce long, sustained energy that will power a lot of our endurance activity. The aerobic system is also powerful as a tool for recovering from some of the other training that you will be doing.

We'll use the aerobic system on our regeneration days to create bloodflow or "flush out" the body. That way, the cells open up so that we can fuel them with pre- and post-workout nutrition, and they'll be available to work even harder on power and strength days. Sometimes there's nothing better than getting a nice, light flush that doesn't beat up your body—a workout that gives you a great sweat plus some volume and distance that serve as a basis for long-term tissue tolerance endurance and recovery.

The aerobic system is important because it improves the mitochondrial and capillary density deep within our muscles. Mitochondria are your body's energy-producing factories. Aerobic work helps place them in locations convenient to the muscles so that they can produce energy and get it to where it's needed most.

Think of your capillaries, or small blood vessels, as a road network that delivers raw materials and gets rid of mitochondrial waste products. Aerobic work helps your capillaries function in the most efficient manner. This is a great reward of cardio: It makes your body more efficient at all levels—in the production of energy, as well as in the import and export of raw materials. With training, your aerobic system can be incredibly efficient at producing sustained energy, and it can also function as one of your most critically important recovery tools.

In this program, we'll operate at times in the "aerobic zone," which means anything below your threshold. To calculate, we'll use the simple, familiar formula of 220 minus your age. If you are 40 years old, that threshold would be 220 minus 40, or 180 beats per minute. Multiply that number by approximately 0.75 to establish your aerobic base, which would be 135. We'll work in your aerobic zone on regeneration days. It should feel relatively easy compared with some of the other training you'll be doing, but it's critical that you understand the boundaries of your zone so that you don't slide into some of the other energy systems, which can lead to overtraining. Be disciplined, and stay under the speed limit.

The lactate power system operates for between 5 seconds and 2 minutes. It does an effective job of producing power for a sustained period, without a heavy reliance on oxygen. But because it uses stored energy in the cells and doesn't rely as much on oxygen, it produces a tremendous amount of waste product.

If your aerobic system is a low-emission Toyota Camry, then your lactate system is a high-emission racecar. The legs and lungs tend to burn as the waste products (such as increased hydrogen ions, which increase the acidity of your blood, sometimes referred to as lactic acid) accumulate and your blood's acidity increases. This is what we perceive as a grueling workout that requires a lot of mental toughness.

These waste products are mainly the result of hydrogen ions and lactate given off as waste products from this system. But this lactate system develops both lactate power and lactate strength, which is your capacity to do intense work. We'll use both of these mechanisms to improve our *anaerobic* or *lactate threshold*, the capacity to do high-intensity work for up to 5-minute intervals. We'll alternate intervals of recovery time to create workouts of up to an hour long.

The lactate threshold may be one of the most important variables in endurance training. We're all familiar with the term *max VO$_2$*, a measure of the amount of oxygen an athlete can take in and process during exercise per unit time. Elite endurance athletes such as Lance Armstrong have a very high max VO$_2$, which is measured in milliliters of oxygen used per kilogram of body mass per minute.

Max VO$_2$ is an important number, but it is not the most critical one. The lactate threshold, which can also be measured like max VO$_2$ but is generally 75 to 90 percent of the max, is what determines when your body will leave its efficient aerobic system and move into the less efficient, yet powerful lactate system. The closer your lactate threshold is to max the better. If your lactate threshold is too far apart from your max VO$_2$, it could make it difficult to achieve your potential as an endurance athlete. Once we hit the lac-

(continued on page 48)

FIND YOUR HEART RATE TRAINING ZONES

By Paul Robbins

If you are a novice endurance athlete or new to the concept of heart rate training, do this "stage training system" prior to following the Core Performance Endurance Energy System Development guidelines. It will help you better establish your base and define your specific heart rate zones.

Stage training is for people who don't have access to a VO_2 analyzer to determine their max VO_2 and anaerobic/lactate threshold. It will allow you to continually adjust and refine your 220-minus-age foundation and your corresponding heart rate values.

STAGE 1:
CREATING AN AEROBIC BASE

You'll use this phase of training for the first of your three heart rate zones. The Stage 1 heart rate zone is 60 to 70 percent of your 220-minus-age heart rate. It should be low enough to ensure that you are in an aerobic state. You'll use this zone during your regeneration days, as well as during the recovery period of your strength and power days. If you are 40 years old, your Stage 1 would be 108 to 126 beats per minute (BPM).

As a novice endurance athlete, you should be able to maintain your Stage 1 heart rate for at least 30 minutes, two or three times per week, which you will accomplish on regeneration days. An example might be walking at a relatively modest speed of 3 miles per hour. This should be a light workout. If it's too easy, ramp up the requirements by adding 5 beats to the zone. Using our 40-year-old example, you would tweak your Stage 1 heart rate zone to 113 to 131 BPM. If Stage 1 is too difficult, reduce it by 5 beats. In this case, our 40-year-old would be at 103 to 121.

At this point, it doesn't matter what exercise equipment you use because you are simply trying to build an aerobic base. Don't feel limited to gym equipment. If you'd rather do your ESD work by walking up hills, jogging, biking, or even swimming, then by all means, go for it. You should, however, purchase a heart rate monitor. (For information on specific products and recommendations, please visit www.coreperformance.com/endurance.)

STAGE 2:
INTRODUCTION TO
INTERVAL TRAINING

Now, you'll build both cardio and leg strength. Stage 2 is an introduction to interval training. Begin with a warmup in Stage 1 for 10 minutes, and then do a 3-minute interval in Stage 2.

To determine your Stage 2 heart rate zone, take 80 to 85 percent of the 220-minus-age formula. Using our 40-year-old example, this would be 144 to 153 beats per minute. Use the formula first but then adjust it if it's too easy or too hard. This zone should be 5 to 10 percent above your adjusted Stage 1 zone. Once your heart rate hits the top of that zone, maintain it for the remainder of the 3-minute interval. It might take just 45 seconds to reach your target heart rate, which means you'll only be at the top end for 2 minutes and 15 seconds before you reduce the workload—either through decreasing the speed or the angle of incline—and return to Stage 1.

Again, it doesn't matter what type of cardiovascular exercise you are doing; just be sure to increase the workload to get your heart rate up to the top of Stage 2. It also doesn't matter whether you use speed or incline to reach Stage 2, because at this point you will determine workload by heart rate.

After finishing the 3-minute interval, return to Stage 1 for 5 minutes. Repeat this sequence (3 minutes in Stage 2, 5 minutes in Stage 1) based on the amount of time you have. The most important part of the interval is to recover back to Stage 1 between intervals in Stage 2. Recovery enables you to repeat the intervals. If your heart rate does not recover, you need to continue working on your aerobic base.

You'll probably need to make adjustments to your target heart rates during the first few training sessions. How hard was it to reach Stage 2? If you couldn't get to what you thought would be Stage 2 within 1 minute, decrease the expected heart rate zone by 5 percent. If you reached Stage 2 with no problem, look to increase time in this zone. Go ahead and do another rep, and as you get really fit, this workout may last up to an hour—or for several hours if needed.

If your heart rate goes beyond the predicted zone, but you're able to recover back to Stage 1, it's because either you have not developed an aerobic base or, if you have been working hard, you may be overtraining. Either way, add a couple of beats to the zone and work on increasing the time.

STAGE 3:
FOR POWER WORKOUTS

If you're ready for a greater challenge, proceed to Stage 3, where we'll create a third zone. Now that you have found a Stage 2 zone that works well for you, add 5 percent to the top heart rate to create your Stage 3 zone. This zone starts where Stage 2 left off and ranges 1 to 5 percent above it. You can make adjustments in this as well, going 2 or 3 beats lower or higher if needed.

Your Stage 3 heart rate zone is used in the power workouts, and it should be one that you can maintain for 5 seconds—2 minutes in the latter levels—and repeat 4 to 12 times, based on the level and phase that you are in.

The most important part of Stage 3 is not to make it too ambitious; the goal is to do all the sprints designed for that stage. If your heart rate in the first sprint is too high, your final sprints will have poor form, which could lead to injury or burnout.

It is best to try all the sprints at your adjusted Stage 3 heart rate zone. If the last sprint is easy, add 1 to 2 beats to the next workout.

Paul Robbins is the metabolic specialist for the Athletes' Performance Institutes.

tate threshold, it's only a matter of time before we hit the wall.

Our goal in training for lactate power and capacity is to elevate the lactate threshold number, the milliliters of oxygen used per kilogram of body mass per minute, raising it from what today might be around 40 up into the 50s. By elevating your lactate threshold, you create a far greater buffer zone, so you can train longer in your aerobic zone at higher intensities and speeds. You'll have far greater leeway before you run into the dangerous lactate threshold.

Let's imagine two endurance runners in a race. The first has a respectable max VO_2 of 60 but a lactate threshold of 40. The second runner, his identical twin, has a max VO_2 that's lower (55) but a lactate threshold of 50. I'll put my money on the second twin, the one with the higher lactate threshold. He has more room in his energy system to work harder before his body enters the lactate system.

Don't get me wrong; at times, the lactate system can be your friend. It will power you on long climbs, aggressive attacks, or the big sprint at the end of the run. The better trained you are within the lactate system, the more rapidly your body will recover from these intense bursts that spew off waste products, which the aerobic system will gobble up and recycle for pure energy. You'll get back into the aerobic zone ready for even more explosive lactate-producing bursts.

That's a powerful weapon to have in your racing arsenal.

Lesser-trained athletes, however—those who ignore training the lactate threshold—might have only one or two bursts before their bodies are completely exhausted. That won't be the case if you work this system. Everyone gets tired, but people who are well-trained recover faster and can deliver high power (wattage) output repeatedly. Your ability to power through a series of lactate bursts is a mark of excellent training and conditioning.

It's not a matter of whether you'll grow tired—you will. But you'll recover faster, enabling you to do more high-quality work. We discussed the waste products given off from the lactate system. One man's garbage is another one's treasure, and this is the great synergy between systems. Your well-developed infrastructure of mitochondrial factories and capillary delivery systems will use lactate system waste products for energy. It transports them readily out of your bloodstream and converts them to powerful, sustained energy for your aerobic system. The upshot? You'll feel less sore, and you'll be able to extend your workout or race for a longer time. You will have power on demand.

Think about this as we get into our interval and lactate training. As we ask you to undergo intense bouts of work that produce lactate and challenge your every system and mental will. We'll also ask you to then decrease the intensity but still stay active, allowing your heart rate to recover and your aerobic system to capture the waste products, turn them into energy, and clear your system so you again can withstand more intense bursts. This is why we create intervals of hard-to-easy to maximize the efficiency of your body's systems. It helps you get the most from training.

Be aware that there is more than one energy system to go out and work every day. Too often, athletes overtrain the system they like to work, which for most is the aerobic system. As a result, they neglect to work the lactate system—the most critical factor in the training methods that will help us improve our lactate threshold. This mistaken approach is like doing the same weight training routine every day and wondering why you don't see much improvement in your strength or power. Contrast that with the progressive and periodized CPE plan, which changes up exercises, sets, reps, days per week, and other variables to achieve great gains.

Before starting the ESD portion of the program, you'll need to create heart rate training "zones." You can do this with a VO_2 analyzer, which you can find at many fitness centers, or you can use the familiar formula of 220 minus your age.

When using this scale, you will need to make adjustments. The formula is based

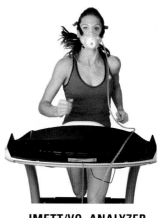

IMETT/VO$_2$ ANALYZER

on a wide range, and most fit individuals don't fit the norm. To create a more personalized training regimen, we'll create a workout of three training stages. After all, to create a balanced cardio or ESD program, you have to not only define the heart rate zones but also adjust them to fit your fitness level and goals. The stage training system on pages 46 and 47, "Find Your Heart Rate Training Zones," was created by Paul Robbins, the Athletes' Performance Institute metabolic specialist, and it will help you create your zones and establish a strong aerobic base.

CHAPTER 5 SUMMARY: Unlike traditional cardio work, Energy System Development focuses on quality, not quantity, and trains the alactate, lactate, and aerobic systems. ESD improves the function of the entire cardiovascular system while building endurance and helping the body tap into new energy levels.

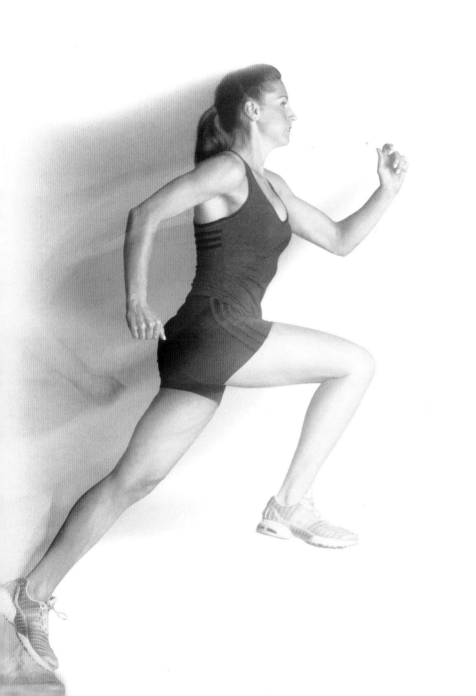

CHAPTER 6

REGENERATION

As an endurance athlete, you take great pride in being able to put forth an all-out effort, all the time. This is a dangerous philosophy because it can lead to injury. At the very least, it's an ineffective way to improve performance.

It's impossible to go all-out all the time. You need some time to recover, a process I call regeneration. Recovery is the limiting factor in performance training, especially for endurance athletes. If you could recover immediately, you could get right back out there and ride, run, or swim longer and faster. You could do it again and again, with no ceiling to your performance level.

This is impossible, of course. You can't continue to go harder and harder without giving your body time to adapt from the training stimulus. Look at this regeneration timeframe as the equivalent of recharging your batteries or refueling your tank. If you recognize and follow this simple formula, you will dramatically increase performance.

WORK + REST = SUCCESS

The things you do at rest are just as important as the work you perform. If you focus on having high-quality rest and regeneration, you'll be able to get more return on investment from every step or minute of your workout.

You're probably already living this concept in other aspects of your life. After all, we could work longer and, in theory, accomplish more if we did not sleep. But we have a

GETTING ENOUGH SLEEP
By Scott Peltin

What if I told you that there was a magic pill that could slow the aging process, increase your energy level, improve your overall health, reduce your risk of premature death, enhance your immune system, make you more mentally alert, and improve your physical and mental performance. Would you believe me? What if I told you that you take it every night, but you may not take enough of it?

This magic pill *does* exist. It's called sleep.

Getting proper nutrition is crucial, but if you eat a bad meal or even skip a meal, you rarely feel like you're ready to collapse. Regular exercise is paramount, but if you skip a workout, it doesn't weaken your immune system, decrease your mental clarity, or destroy your mood.

Sleep, on the other hand, is the foundation of everything we do. It allows us to rebuild our bodies, to replenish our chemical stores, and to have the alertness to function throughout the day.

In 2001, the National Sleep Foundation performed its famous Sleep in America survey, determining that 63 percent of adults get less than the recommended 8 hours of sleep per night, and 31 percent get less than 7 hours. More than 40 percent of adult Americans reported having trouble staying awake during the day.

Sleep deprivation can interfere with memory, energy levels, mental abilities, and mood. In a study conducted by the University of Chicago Medical Center in 1999, researchers found that the condition drastically affects the body's ability to metabolize glucose, leading to

symptoms that mimic early-stage diabetes.

Sleep deprivation also can contribute to heart disease, diabetes, obesity, and cancer. Without sleep, you simply cannot function at your best. Sleep debt undermines your ability to eat healthfully and exercise. When the brain is exhausted, it doesn't know whether it is sleep-deprived or starving for glucose. So its natural response is to crave sugar. This is why you have so many late-night cravings when you're tired. When you're low on energy, your brain wants to conserve energy, so motivation to exercise is greatly reduced.

Sleep occurs in stages, each with a different EEG (brain wave) pattern. While sleep researchers may classify sleep into many stages, there are just two basic forms of sleep: slow much more efficient, higher quality of work if we sleep 6 to 8 hours. We also could work more hours over the course of a year if we didn't take vacations. Yet most of us discover that we're far more productive if we schedule some time to relax and recharge.

This regeneration plan will increase energy, boost your immune system, and help

wave sleep (SWS) and rapid eye movement (REM) sleep.

As we age, less of our sleep is REM sleep. REM sleep is where dreams occur but our muscles are inactive. SWS sleep is actually four different stages, and it's important for many of the restorative functions of sleep.

During the first deep sleep of the night, the greatest amount of growth hormone is secreted to help the body repair the damage that has occurred throughout the day. This may be why phone calls that occur within the first hour of falling asleep seem to leave you so worn out the following day.

Early researchers believed that sleep cycles occurred every 90 minutes and that therefore, healthy sleep should fit into these 90-minute blocks. Newer sleep research indicates that

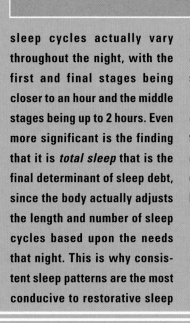

PHYSICAL ACTIVITY

PROPER NUTRITION

ADEQUATE SLEEP

sleep cycles actually vary throughout the night, with the first and final stages being closer to an hour and the middle stages being up to 2 hours. Even more significant is the finding that it is *total sleep* that is the final determinant of sleep debt, since the body actually adjusts the length and number of sleep cycles based upon the needs that night. This is why consistent sleep patterns are the most conducive to restorative sleep

and inconsistent sleep patterns are the most likely to lead to sleep deprivation.

Proper sleep is paramount for an endurance athlete, not only to recover and regenerate but also to be prepared for the next day. It's by far the easiest way to boost performance.

Scott Peltin is a founding partner of Tignum AG, a performance institute for corporate leaders and a strategic partner of Athletes' Performance Institutes.

you get the most return out of each training session, which ultimately will improve your performance. Regeneration will improve your hormone profile, decrease inflammation, and improve tissue quality, thus decreasing the number of overuse injuries you may experience.

The regeneration strategy is not just one unit; it permeates the entire Core Performance Endurance system, whether we're talking about performance planning, nutrition, vacations, family time, or hobbies. In the United States, we've developed such a nose-to-the-grindstone mentality when it comes to work that we've become inefficient. We work so hard, with so little time to recover, that our productivity suffers, and ultimately, we break down. We want to be more efficient and enjoy all aspects of our lives more. Regeneration helps that happen.

It's easy to see the regeneration concept at work in Europe, where businesses close for daily siestas and people typically receive 6 weeks of vacation a year. You might not agree with the practical aspects of that, but it's undeniable that such recovery periods contribute to healthier, more energized employees.

Regeneration starts with how we plan our training. We'll schedule regeneration into each day, and we'll schedule regeneration days during the course of the week. In addition to keeping a regeneration mindset and

doing specific "regen" workouts to improve the quality of your tissue, you'll see the concept of regeneration built into the nutrition program as well.

Think of regeneration in terms of *active* regeneration and *passive* regeneration.

Active regeneration consists of easy aerobic activity, such as long, easy rides on the bike or a swim. The idea here is to avoid pounding and huge energy expenditure.

Passive regeneration involves such activities as massages and hot and cold contrasts (more on those in a minute). But passive regeneration is also a mindset, the idea that we're working constantly to become better, even when we're not working out. This philosophy includes getting proper sleep—even taking naps—and planning ahead to make the most of time. It also involves taking vacations and enjoying leisure pursuits. Of course, your endurance activity might be your leisure pursuit, but you also need things that aren't as taxing on the body.

The regeneration unit requires some inexpensive items: a foam roll and an 8-foot length of rope. The roll is an 18-inch-long roll of tightly packed foam that's roughly 5 inches in diameter. On regeneration days, you'll rotate and roll your hamstrings, quadriceps, back, lats, and hips over the foam roll.

The foam roll routine is like a massage. It uses deep compression to help roll out the muscle spasms that develop over time. The compression overstimulates the nerves, which signals the muscle spasm to shut off. This allows the muscles to relax and loosen up, gets the blood and lymphatic system flowing, and helps the body recover. Think of your body as clay. The roll softens up the clay, so you can remold it into something more pliable and functional.

As we've said before, tissue is like a rubber band. Our goal is to keep it supple and elastic. Unfortunately, it tends to get knotted up with spasms over time. If you put 20 knots into a rubber band, it's the same rubber band, but it doesn't store nearly as much energy. More stress goes into a few parts of the rubber band instead of dispersing throughout the band. The goal with our self-massage and our isolative and static stretching (to be discussed shortly) is to undo the knots and spasms. Once we get those worked out, we need to address them daily and weekly to make sure that no more knots accumulate. It takes consistent, proactive maintenance. Think of your tissue the way you might a long-haired dog. If you don't brush the dog every day, he'll end up matted, and your only alternative will be to have him shaved. Let's not do the equivalent to our tissue.

You'll probably enjoy the foam-roll routine—everyone likes massages. Still, there will be some uncomfortable moments, as there are with a professional massage. Once you're past the first few weeks, though, it will become considerably easier and more comfortable. The foam roll is a great barometer of the quality of your muscle and connective tissue. The better it feels, and the less it hurts, the higher the quality of your tissue.

Feel free to work with the foam roll on non-regeneration days; it's easy to do while watching television. Don't limit yourself to the areas targeted in this program. Use it anywhere you feel tight and in need of a massage. Foam rolls are inexpensive and available at www.coreperformance.com/endurance.

The other component of the regeneration unit is active-isolated stretching (AIS), developed by Aaron Mattes. This will require an 8- to 10-foot length of rope, about the thickness of jump rope. You can go to a home improvement store and have a length cut off for just a few dollars, or you can check out the ropes at www.coreperformance.com/endurance.

You'll wrap the rope around one foot at a time and perform a series of moves that will reprogram your muscles to contract and relax through new ranges of motion. You won't hold stretches for 10 to 30 seconds, as in traditional stretching, because that doesn't require your body to actively reprogram itself for new ranges of motion.

Instead, you'll use the rope to gently assist the muscle's range of motion about 10 to 20 percent farther than your body would ordinarily allow. You're going to exhale during the assistance portion, releasing tension and getting a deeper stretch. Finally, you'll pull your leg back to the starting position.

The key is that you're reprogramming your brain. Say that you're doing a hamstring stretch. You're lying on your back, with a rope wrapped around one leg. First, you pull your toe up toward your shin. Then you squeeze, or "fire," your quadriceps, hip flexors, and abs. As you squeeze, they contract, and your hamstrings automatically relax. That enables you to gently assist with the rope to pull your hamstrings into a slightly deeper stretch, helping to reprogram your brain and muscles for that new range of motion.

YOUR SLEEP NUMBER

So, how do you improve quality of sleep? Michael J. Breus, author of *Good Night: The Sleep Doctor's 4-Week Program to Better Sleep and Better Health* and a friend of Athletes' Performance Institutes, has some specific recommendations for endurance athletes.

First, determine your "sleep number." Most endurance athletes have a tendency to ignore or reduce sleep in lieu of training time, thus decreasing total sleep time. This is not a good idea. Recovery from muscle strain occurs during sleep; sleep is not just a time for rest. People need to determine exactly how much sleep they will need each night to feel refreshed the next day.

Once you have that number, determine when you must wake up. Then work backward to determine your bedtime, based on how you feel each morning. Try going to bed at 10 p.m. and rate your sleepiness in the morning on a scale of 1 to 10, with 1 being not sleepy and 10 very sleepy. Once you get to 4, you're getting close to your sleep number and can tweak accordingly.

Many endurance athletes don't give themselves sufficient time to relax before bed. Since they train so much of the day, they save evenings for chores, emotionally charged family issues, and so on.

Instead, create what I call a "power-down hour" where, for the hour prior to sleep, you spend 30 minutes doing low-key household chores such as dishes or laundry—certainly nothing as ambitious as scrubbing floors. Allot 15 minutes to change into bedclothes and for personal hygiene and the final 15 minutes for meditation, reading, relaxation, and stretching.

Finally, pay attention to your body's need for sleep. Learn the difference between fatigue, which is characterized by muscle soreness and feeling worn out, and sleepiness, where your eyelids are heavy, and you actually catch yourself falling asleep.

It's important to remember to assist with the rope only at the very end of the motion. Exhale and release the tension from your body and mind.

There are two other key components to regeneration: sleep and "contrasts."

At our Athletes' Performance Institutes, we have athletes alternate between sitting for 3 to 5 minutes in a hot tub and 1 minute to 3 minutes in a 55°F "cold plunge" tub. When done after a workout, the contrasts stimulate muscle recovery with little effort. The cold therapy, in particular, decreases the natural post-workout inflammation in our muscles, and it is often used alone for 6 to 15 minutes immediately after a workout.

When you enter the warm water, the blood flows out to your skin and limbs to increase the surface area to dissipate heat—just as your skin flushes when exercising in the heat. The cold does the opposite, pulling blood away from the skin and limbs and toward the heart, not unlike what happens when your fingers turn blue in extreme cold. This contrast between the hot and cold simulates exercise by circulating blood through your body, but without spending energy.

Hot and cold contrasts force your blood to move fast, from your trunk to your skin and back again. That's a good thing in and of itself. But when you do it immediately after a workout, you stimulate bloodflow and muscle recovery with hardly any effort. (Resistance exercise and running create tiny microtears in muscle fibers, which your body repairs in between workouts, leaving your muscles ready to adapt to further training.)

You don't need access to a hot tub or a cold plunge; you can get the same effect in the shower by switching between hot and cold settings.

CHAPTER 6 SUMMARY: It's impossible to go all-out all the time. One of the key elements to achieving optimal performance is the notion of recovery or *regeneration.* By taking measures to help your body recover, you'll be better positioned to thrive during your next workout. These measures include proper planning, nutrition, sleep, active-isolated stretching, foam roll work, and hot and cold contrasts.

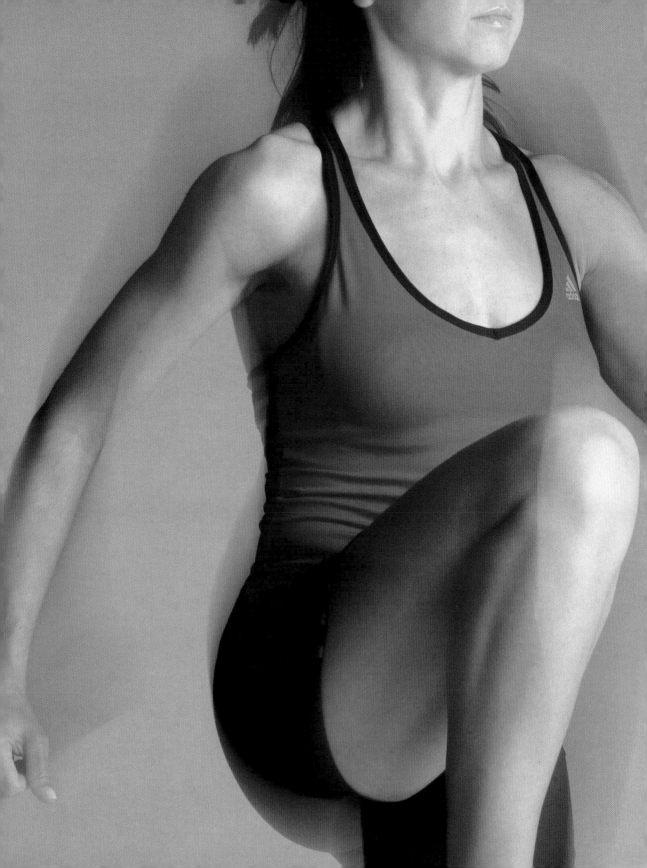

PART 3

CORE ENDURANCE NUTRITION

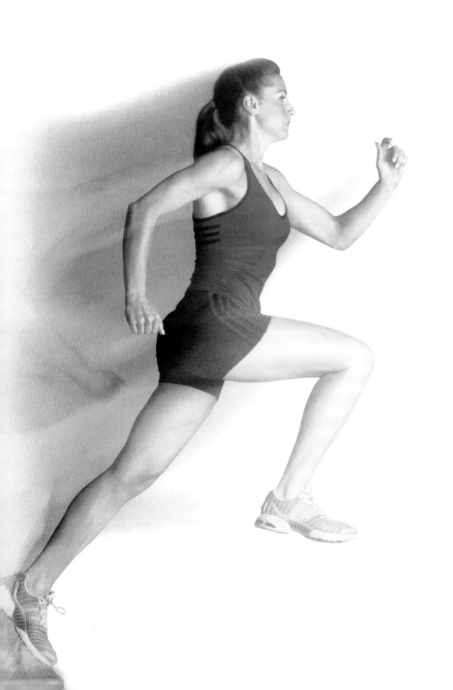

CHAPTER 7

EAT TO PERFORM

n my previous two books, *Core Performance* and *Core Performance Essentials*, I spent a lot of time showing readers the basics of nutrition. If you're reading this book, you probably have a solid base of nutritional knowledge. But what I've discovered in working with endurance athletes, even those at the elite level, is that they can still use some easy-to-follow strategies to fuel their bodies for optimum performance.

In fact, many endurance athletes run themselves into the ground. Too often, endurance athletes see food as the enemy, not as a vital component to high performance. They believe food will add pounds to their frames and seconds to their times. Some might not even see the correlation between food and their training and performance. Others figure they burn so many calories training that they can consume pretty much whatever they want.

That thinking could not be more erroneous. Would you run a high-performance engine without making sure it's properly fueled and lubricated with the best available products? If you did, you wouldn't get the most out of the engine, and you would greatly increase the chance of a breakdown.

Best-case scenario, you still wouldn't be getting the most out of it.

If you're not fueling your body properly, you're sabotaging that high-performance engine you've worked so hard to create through training. In fact, if you've ignored nutrition up until this point, you've probably reached only a fraction of your potential.

Too often, I see endurance athletes who roll out of bed—early, of course, to begin their training—but don't eat anything. When they do eat, they stay away from carbohydrates, the very fuel they need to perform well. Those popular low-carb diets are meant for sedentary people who spend their lives behind a desk and in front of the television (though even for them, I'd recommend a more balanced, healthy approach).

Many endurance athletes, especially those at the elite level, are so obsessed with weight and calories that they're almost like jockeys in horse racing. Now, I recognize the athleticism that jockeys must have, but the endurance athlete is more like the horse. If you don't fuel your body properly, you're depriving it of essential nutrients and decreasing energy levels, which is going to have a negative effect on your training and performance.

Not only that, but these poor nutritional habits place you on a downward spiral that will weaken your bone density and leave you more susceptible to injury and illness.

There's no way you can improve your performance unless you recognize that half of the formula is eating properly. Nutrition not only fuels your body for every training session, it also ensures proper recovery. Fueling your body will increase your energy levels and enhance the quality of your training, enabling you to maximize each of your training days and competitions.

Proper diet wards off disease, allowing you to maximize the ultimate goal of training: your health. Eating right also decreases inflammation that contributes to muscle pain, joint discomfort, and overuse injuries.

If you were to read a product label that promised everything listed in the two previous paragraphs, you'd rush to buy it. Fortunately, you already have, in the form of this book.

You need to view nutrition as your workout partner, an essential tool to optimize your health, training, and performance. So many people view food either with fear ("it will make me fat") or with love ("I live to eat"). We don't want to be afraid of food, nor do we want to live to eat. Instead, we should *eat to live*. Let's look at food more objectively, as a potentially powerful means to fuel performance.

As an endurance athlete, you've dedicated a significant chunk of your life to strengthening, stretching, and otherwise training to achieve a balanced body. But

THE FEMALE ATHLETE TRIAD
By Amanda Carlson, MS, RD

By following the Core Performance Endurance nutrition plan, your body will become lean and efficient. After all, excess body fat hinders performance and quality of life.

That said, there's a fine line to walk between being lean and efficient and becoming *too* lean. With female endurance athletes, especially those in their late teens and early twenties, we sometimes see what's known as the "female athlete triad," an obsession with body weight that becomes dangerous and leads to serious health consequences. The female athlete triad is a three-part progression, from disordered eating to amenorrhea to osteoporosis: An athlete restricts calories to reduce body fat to the point where she becomes "amenorrheic"—she stops menstruating. When that occurs, hormones change, and the body begins to break down bones.

There's a dangerous notion that losing a normal menstrual period for only a short time is acceptable. In truth, the loss of a normal menstrual period means that the body is severely out of balance.

These young women come to believe that the leaner they are, the better they will perform. Therefore, they start to seriously restrict their caloric intake and slip into patterns of disordered eating or even a full-blown eating disorder. There are instances of women running 15 miles a day on just 1,500 calories and thinking they're eating enough!

If you restrict caloric intake too much, your performance will suffer. What these young women might perceive as a few extra calories that could boost body fat may actually help their performance.

We want to give you the solutions to stay lean, be in great health, and perform at a high level. You can have it all. So many female athletes don't realize the damage they're doing to their bodies.

We've seen bone scans on female endurance athletes who have become so lean that they're showing signs of osteoporosis at the age of 30. Their bodies' systems no longer adapt to the demands of training. Instead, they get into a downward spiral of injury, illness, and long-term absences from their beloved endurance sports. All this is in addition to the long-term health consequences of early-onset osteoporosis and the possibility of being unable to bear children. Athletes in their twenties often don't consider these long-term repercussions, which really are not that far off.

When it comes to nutrition, listen to your body, and provide it with the fuel it needs to live, train, and thrive. What you might perceive as a few extra pounds actually will help your performance and ensure good health in the future.

Amanda Carlson, MS, RD, is director of performance nutrition for the Athletes' Performance Institutes.

what does that supposedly balanced body look like on the inside? There are many amazing athletes who, on the surface, are picture-perfect models of bodies in balance. Inside, however, they're on the brink of collapse. They're the equivalent of a 3-year-old Corvette that's never had an oil change or a fluid check.

If you don't give your body the fuel it needs, it becomes catabolic, drawing fuel from your lean muscle—the very thing you've worked so hard to create. In the catabolic state, muscles are constantly running on fumes. When the body has not been given the proper fuel it needs to run or recover, its ability to take on the stress of daily life and training becomes increasingly compromised, and it never has the chance to fully heal. When your body does not have the chance to recover, it enters a state of imbalance and becomes overtrained. Your resting heart rate will increase, and you will have decreases in endurance and power, the very things you're training to improve.

This unbalanced state makes your body more susceptible to sickness, fatigue, depression, inflammation, injury, and loss of competitive fire, and it diminishes performance.

A proper nutrition program is one of the most effective tools to put your body back into balance after training. By getting enough calories and nutrients, you'll enable your body to run efficiently and your energy stores to remain full.

Even if you think you're eating properly right now, I guarantee that the following pages will show you ways to eat better and improve performance. Nutrition should be used as a way to enhance your health, your energy, and your performance. Proper post-workout nutrition is essential. It restores your body's hormonal equilibrium and jump-starts repair and recovery, assuming the rest of your nutrition program is effective. Almost all of the endurance athletes I see do not know how to properly fuel themselves for day-to-day living, let alone before and after workouts.

Endurance athletes are planners. They will meticulously plan their training sessions and schedule their day to the minute, but then they may have no idea what they are going to eat for their next meal or snack. Often, I'll ask an endurance athlete what he consumes after a competition or workout, and he'll give me a puzzled look. *The race is over. I don't feel like having anything. Maybe a bottle of water. Or a beer!*

In short, proper nutrition is the easiest and most effective way to enhance your health and performance. That's why we're going to discuss nutrition before we go into the specifics of the Core Performance Endurance training methods. If you never read the training portion of this book and just apply what you learn in this section, I guarantee you'll still see improvement. If you skip this section of the book, continue to follow your existing eating habits, and apply our training methods, your progress will be only a fraction of what it would be if you incorporated healthy eating.

So, before we learn the workout system, let's lay a solid foundation by adopting some new nutrition habits. They'll fuel your performance, save you time and money, and improve the quality of your life.

We're going to keep this easy, breaking nutrition down into five simple strategies, along with the following chapter on supplementation. If you can master these strategies, combined with our CPE workout program, you'll be in phenomenal shape and you'll achieve a state of balance—inside and out.

ENDURANCE NUTRITION STRATEGY #1: FUEL UP WITH CARBS

Popular diets have conditioned people to believe that carbohydrates must be avoided at all costs. Just as the anti-fat trend of the 1980s gave fats a bad name, today, carbs have been unfairly labeled as the enemy.

Everything is classified into three nutrient groups—carbs, protein, and fat—and if we neglect any of the three, we're depriving the body of important nutrients it needs to live. Following a low-carb diet is especially dangerous for endurance athletes, who need carbs to thrive in their sports.

Carbs are our primary source of fuel. They provide energy for muscle function and act as the primary fuel for the brain. When you don't take in enough carbs, your body does not run efficiently or effectively. As a result, you don't have high-quality workouts, and your body never recovers properly. But if you eat the right types of carbs at the right time, it allows you to train harder and longer, which stimulates performance.

Think of carbs as the fuel for your body's gas tank. When consumed in the proper amounts, carbs are used for energy and stored in the liver and the muscles for future energy needs. If you eat too many carbs, they will overflow the gas tank and be stored as fat. But if you don't eat enough carbs, you'll run out of fuel during your workouts, and that will lead to decreased performance.

You need to fuel your body based on the size of your gas tank. As an endurance athlete, you have much higher fuel needs than someone who sits behind a desk all day and doesn't exercise. You're working out regularly, driving that "car," and you burn a lot of fuel—a lot of carbs. As your training increases and decreases over the course of a week, month, or year, so should your carbohydrate intake. However, don't lump yourself in with inactive folks. Low-carb diets are not for you!

Not all carbs are created equal, of course. When planning meals, we want to avoid processed carbs, such as white breads, pastas, and baked goods. They provide little nutritional value and are converted quickly to sugar and easily stored as fat.

Instead, we want to include fruits, vegetables, and whole grains because of their fiber and nutrient density. Your meals should consist mostly of colorful, high-fiber vegetables and grains, which contain powerful vitamins and antioxidants that help to protect the body from the cell-damaging effects of free radicals. If you opt for pasta or couscous, choose the whole wheat option. If you reach for rice, opt for brown rice.

When in doubt, follow the advice of Amanda Carlson, the director of performance nutrition at Athletes' Peformance, and "come back to earth." When given a choice between something processed and something more natural, go with the non-processed option.

It's important to include carbs in your pre-run or pre-workout meal and in your postrun/post-workout meal. Later in this chapter, I will discuss how to use the glycemic index for health and for sports. Generally speaking, choose slower-digesting carbs during the day and before your activity and include more processed carbs when you need quick energy, such as during or after workouts.

So, what quantity of carbs do you need? Don't make the mistake of trying to look at it as a percentage of your caloric intake; many endurance athletes have restricted their intake. Instead, go with 2 to 4 grams of carbohydrates per pound of body weight per day.

Consuming the recommended amount of carbs each day will ensure that you have optimal fuel stores for training and also help bring your body into balance. An easy way to measure portion size is to use your fist as a guide. Generally speaking, include a fist-size portion of carbs at most of your meals. If you are in an intense training phase, or this

NEGATIVE EFFECTS OF A LOW-CARB DIET

Need more convincing? A low-carb diet is like taking a sponge and wringing the water out. You'll lose the water weight, but as soon as you eat carbs again—and you will at some point, because you need energy to function, and you can only go so long without them—the sponge is going to fill up with water.

Losing water weight is especially dangerous for endurance athletes. For each gram of carbs we store, we also put away 3 grams of water, which is critical to staying hydrated during strenuous activity.

THE GLYCEMIC INDEX

One way to separate good carbs from bad is through the glycemic index, a measure of how a single food will raise your blood glucose level. A food that's highly glycemic will be digested quickly and is absorbed immediately, sending your blood sugar level sky-high. The problem is that you crash quickly and end up feeling sluggish.

If you eat the same portion of a low-glycemic food, your body has to work harder to break it down. The benefit is that the sugar from the food will be released into the bloodstream more slowly, giving you steady energy over a longer period.

This is the difference between eating a low-glycemic food, such as green peas, and a high-glycemic food, such as a doughnut. You already know that the peas are better than the doughnut, but it's not just because the peas will give you nutrients, and the doughnut will add to your midsection. They also have radically different short-term effects on your energy levels, moods, and performance.

Generally speaking, the lower the number on the glycemic index, the more natural the food will be. Your body has to do the work to get the nutrients out of these foods, and that's good, because that gradual release helps regulate blood sugar. Look for natural foods that have more color and fiber, because those foods control appetite, have more nutrients, and improve your cardiovascular system.

By controlling your blood sugar, you're regulating the hormone insulin. If you're constantly jacking up your blood sugar by eating only high-glycemic foods, you create a vicious cycle that results in increased calorie consumption and body fat levels, obesity, and perhaps even diabetes.

GLYCEMIC INDEX OF POPULAR FOODS

LOW	MODERATE	HIGH
Sweet potatoes	Mashed potatoes	Baked potatoes
Yams	Sweet corn	Doughnuts
Green peas	Bananas	Waffles
Black beans	Cantaloupe	Bagels
Oatmeal (not instant)	Pineapple	Raisin bran
Peaches	Hamburger buns	Graham crackers
Oranges	Muffins	Pretzels
Apples	Cheese pizza	Corn chips
Grapefruit	Oatmeal cookies	Watermelon

is your post-training meal, make the portion the size of two fists.

The bottom line is that most endurance athletes do not consume enough carbs. If you've been cutting back on your carbs, I promise that if you start consuming the proper amount of this crucial nutrient, your performance will increase immediately.

PERFORMANCE POINTS:
- Carbs are critical for fueling endurance athletes.

- Choose lower glycemic index carbs that are rich in fiber when planning your meals. (See "The Glycemic Index," on page 67.) Fist-size portions are a good guideline.

- Choose higher glycemic carbs for meals or snacks immediately following your training session—two fists.

- If you choose to eat more processed carbs, consume them during the period after a training session or race.

IS THE GLYCEMIC INDEX OVERRATED?

By Amanda Carlson, MS, RD

The glycemic index is a trendy topic. Three years ago, few athletes paid attention to the "GI," which ranks carbs according to their ability to affect blood glucose. These days, most everyone has some idea of what the GI represents—or at least they think they do.

The popular perception is that low-glycemic diets will help people lose weight and reduce the risk of heart disease and diabetes. This notion is based on early studies evaluating the GI of different foods, studies conducted in a controlled environment on subjects who had fasted overnight. The subjects ate a single specific carbohydrate in a prescribed amount and had their blood glucose measured 2 hours later.

In a controlled setting, the low-GI carb is broken down more slowly, which produces a more consistent glucose level. A high-GI carb is just the opposite. It is broken down quickly and causes a spike in blood glucose, followed by a subsequent blood glucose crash. A moderate GI falls somewhere in the middle.

The problem is that such studies don't apply to real life. Breakfast is the only time we eat after fasting, and additional factors such as the length of time the food is cooked, the body's hormones, and any other food (protein or fat) that is eaten in combination with the carbohydrate can alter how the body uses glucose.

One recent study conducted at the University of Southern California found that those who followed a lower-GI diet did not have significantly lower blood glucose levels than those who followed a relatively higher GI-carb diet.

ENDURANCE NUTRITION STRATEGY #2: IMPROVE PERFORMANCE WITH PROTEIN

Many athletes struggle to find the happy medium when it comes to protein. On one hand, there are endurance athletes who have overcompensated when it comes to carbs, believing that carbohydrates are the only nutrient involved in their performance, so they don't think about protein. Then there are folks who follow the dangerous low-carb trend and go overboard on protein.

Protein builds, maintains, and restores muscle. It's responsible for healthy blood cells, key enzymes, and strengthening the immune system. In order to build muscle, protein must be consumed with enough carbohydrate calories to provide the body with energy. Otherwise, your body will tap into the protein for energy. Using protein for energy is inefficient and ineffective when it comes to performance.

Just as endurance athletes have higher

Other studies link *dietary fiber* to a decreased risk of heart disease, diabetes, and obesity. This raises the question of what makes the food healthful—its GI, or the components that rank it low on the glycemic index. In other words, it could be that the food is healthful first and foremost because of its fiber properties. Foods low on the GI are typically higher in fiber. Therefore, many of the studies linking GI to good health may have, in fact, reflected the dietary fiber found in those foods.

I don't mean to knock the glycemic index. It has taught us that not all carbs are created equal. But the GI is not the sole solution to controlling weight, preventing heart disease, or managing diabetes. It's just one piece of the puzzle.

The bottom line is that foods lower on the GI tend to be whole foods, with more nutrients and more fiber.

Rather than obsessing over the GI, choose the least processed form of foods available to you. Don't make things complicated. When choosing carbs, reach for fruits, veggies, beans, and whole grains. When shopping for breads and cereals, look for fiber. If the cereal or bread has 3 or more grams of fiber per serving, go for it. If not, find something else.

Instead of viewing the GI—or any other measuring stick—as the one-stop source for food evaluation, include whole grains, fiber, fruits, vegetables, lean proteins, and healthy fats in your diet. That's a formula that any scientific study will support.

Amanda Carlson, MS, RD, is director of performance nutrition for the Athletes' Performance Institutes.

carbohydrate needs than the average person, they also need more protein. This is especially true of endurance athletes who incorporate strength training into their regimen, as you'll do in the Core Performance Endurance system.

Exercise, especially endurance training, produces a catabolic effect, breaking down precious lean body mass. By consuming adequate protein, both throughout the day and especially after our training sessions, we help our bodies minimize and reverse this breakdown effect and jump-start them on the road to recovery.

As a general rule of thumb, you need to consume between 0.6 and 0.8 gram of protein per pound of body weight. If you weigh, say, 180 pounds, you want to shoot for between 108 and 144 grams of protein per day. Endurance athletes tend to fall on the high side of this scale, so you'll probably want to be closer to 0.8 gram.

This protein will be split up over the course of the day, but it should be included in every meal. Protein helps to stabilize energy and also revs up the metabolism. Your body has to work a little harder to digest protein; therefore, your metabolism gets a jolt each time you eat protein. By including a protein source in each of your meals and your post-workout recovery shake (we'll get to that later), you will easily and effectively satisfy your protein needs.

Here's a good rule of thumb regarding protein: "The less legs, the better." The fewer legs something has—or at least had when it was alive—the better its ratio of protein to healthy fat.

Fish, for instance, have no legs, and fish is a healthy source of protein, assuming that it's not fried. Fish also provides omega-3 and omega-6 fatty acids. The omega-3 fatty acid helps to promote cardiovascular health and decreases inflammation. Chickens have two legs and also are a wonderful source of protein, provided the skin is removed and the meat is not fried.

Meat from four-legged creatures can be good, provided it's a lean cut. Lean red meat is a source of important nutrients such as iron and phosphorus. Lean cuts of pork also are good sources of protein.

Low-fat dairy products provide not only protein but also calcium and vitamin D for strong bones.

When you start to consider how much protein you really need to eat, you may think that it sounds like a lot, but in reality, I'm not asking you to consume half a cow each day. Note how much protein is in these common foods:

- Chicken (4 ounces, skinless, the size of a deck of cards): 35 grams

- Cod or salmon (6 ounces): 40 grams

- Tuna (6 ounces, packed in water): 40 grams

- Lean pork (4 ounces): 35 grams

- Lean red meat (4 ounces): 35 grams

- Reduced-fat tofu (6 ounces): 30 grams

- Cottage cheese (1 cup of 1% fat): 28 grams

- Milk (1 cup of 1% or fat-free): 8 grams

- One egg: 6 grams

- One egg white: 3 grams

We're also going to incorporate post-workout recovery shakes into your routine. Each will contain 20 to 45 grams of protein per serving. If you have one or two shakes a day, along with some combination of poultry and fish for lunch and dinner and a breakfast that includes yogurt or egg whites, you'll easily meet your daily protein goal.

PERFORMANCE POINTS:

- Endurance athletes have high protein needs. Make sure you take in 0.8 gram of protein per pound per day.

- Include lean protein in every meal.

- A "deck of cards" portion of chicken, lean pork, or lean red meat (about 4 ounces) is equivalent to 35 grams of protein.

ENDURANCE NUTRITION STRATEGY #3:
EAT THE RIGHT KIND OF FAT

We need a new word to refer to the nutrient fat. Thanks to the aggressive anti-fat marketing campaigns of the 1980s, most people believe that if you eat fat, you become fat.

There's some truth to that, of course. Not all fat is good, and too much of anything will contribute to additional body fat. But fats are crucial to good health and the makeup of cell membranes. Fats release energy slowly, keeping the body satiated and regulating blood sugar, thus lowering glycemic response to other foods. Good fats provide powerful nutrients for cellular repair of the joints, organs, skin, and hair. Fats, especially those found in fish oil and flaxseed oil, also help with cognitive ability, mental clarity, and memory retention, and they have strong anti-inflammatory properties.

We want to avoid saturated fats, which are usually found in meat and dairy foods and are solid at room temperature. Saturated fats raise serum cholesterol, clog arteries, and pose a risk to the heart.

The easiest way to avoid saturated fats is to limit your intake of whole-fat dairy products and red meat that's marbled and fatty. The only difference between whole milk and skim products is the saturated fat content. When choosing dairy, go with products labeled 1% or below.

We also want to stay away from trans fats, which raise bad (LDL) cholesterol but do not raise good (HDL) cholesterol. Artery-clogging trans fats are found in processed foods such as cookies, crackers, pies, pastries, and margarine. They're also found in fried foods and in smaller quantities in meat

(continued on page 74)

CORE GROCERY LIST

GENERAL SHOPPING TIPS
● Stay focused. ● Go in with a plan. ● Avoid products at the heads of the aisles.
● Watch out at the checkout! ● Explore one new healthy food with each shopping trip.

BAKERY
100% whole wheat bread
(look for fiber)
Pumpernickel bread/products
Sourdough bread/products

CEREAL AISLE
Bran cereal
Kashi cereal (my personal favorite)

CANNED FOODS
Black beans
Fruit, packaged, with no sugar
added (canned in its own juice)
Kidney beans
Navy beans
Pinto beans
Tuna, water-packed

DELI SECTION
*TIP: Avoid deli salads
and fried foods.*
Deli meats, lean and reduced-fat
(turkey, chicken, roast beef, ham)
Hummus
Rotisserie chicken (remove skin
and pat off excess oil)

BAKING, SNACK, AND
CONDIMENT AISLES
Almonds
Canola oil
Enova oil
High-protein meal-replacement
bars
Mustard
Olive oil
Peanut butter, natural

Peanuts
Salad dressing, low-fat
Sunflower seeds
Vinegar, balsamic or red wine
(for salads)

MEAT AND
SEAFOOD AISLES
Chicken, skinless, white meat
Ground beef, 96% fat-free
Red meat and pork, lean
Salmon and other fish
Turkey, white meat

DAIRY SECTION
TIP: Avoid whole-milk products.
Cheese, reduced-fat
Cottage cheese, 1% or fat-free
Juices, 100% juice,
no sugar added
Milk, 1% or fat-free
Yogurt, low-fat, low-sugar

FROZEN FOODS
Fruits
Ice cream, low-fat, low-sugar
Juices, 100% juice, no sugar
added
Kashi waffles
Soy yogurt or ice cream
Vegetables

PRODUCE SECTION
*TIPS: Stock up! Cut and
package produce to eat later.*
Apples, red or green
Apricots
Bananas

Blueberries
Broccoli
Carrots
Cauliflower
Cucumber
Edamame
Grapefruit
Grapes, red
Green beans
Kiwifruit
Oranges
Pears
Romaine lettuce
Spinach
Strawberries
Sweet potatoes
Tofu
Tomatoes

PHARMACY
Antioxidant complex
Calcium (for women)
Fish oil/omega-3 capsules (Udo's
Choice Blend is one good brand)
Multivitamin
Vitamin C (500 mg)
Vitamin E (400 IU)
Whey protein powder

BEVERAGE AISLES
Coffee, regular and decaf
Dry beverages
(such as Crystal Light)
Juices, 100% juice,
no sugar added
Tea, green, white, and black
Water, bottled
Wine, red

SERVING SIZES

Vegetables: 1 cup raw leafy vegetables, ½ cup cooked or raw vegetables, ¾ cup vegetable juice, ½ cup cooked dry beans

Fruits: 1 medium-size fruit (1 medium apple or 1 medium pear), ½ cup canned or chopped fruit, or ¾ cup fruit juice

Breads and Cereals: 1 slice of bread, 1 cup ready-to-eat cereal, ½ cup cooked rice or pasta

Protein: 4 ounces meat (size of a deck of cards), handful of nuts

Fats: 1 tablespoon olive oil, 1 tablespoon Enova oil, 1 tablespoon flaxseed oil, 1 tablespoon fish oil, 2 tablespoons peanut butter

Dairy: 1 cup milk, ½ cup cottage cheese, 1 ounce or slice of cheese

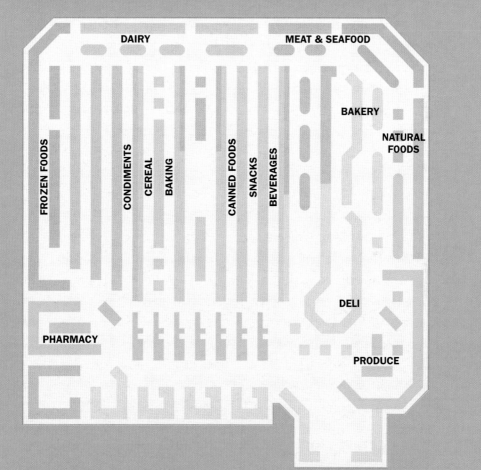

Stay along the perimeter of the store. Avoid the middle aisles, except for the occasional healthy item.

and some dairy products. Thankfully, food manufacturers must now list trans fat amounts on their product labels.

However, even if the label says "no trans fat," there is a chance that there may be some trans fat in the product. If there is less than 0.5 gram of trans fat per serving, the FDA allows the manufacturer to place "no trans fat" onto the package. Yep—the FDA allows the manufacturer to round down. So read the Nutrition Facts label *and* the ingredients list. If the words "hydrogenated" or "fractionated" appear in any of the first four ingredients, the product likely contains trans fats. If you are choosing minimally processed, whole foods, you should not have to worry about trans fats.

The best fats come out of nuts, fish oils, and seeds. Nuts and seeds are a convenient source of protein and fiber, and they stick with you longer than many snacks, helping to control blood sugar and appetite. A handful of nuts every day can lower your risk of heart ailments and Alzheimer's disease and can even be used to lower cholesterol.

Nuts and seeds are unsaturated fats, which do not raise cholesterol levels. The best unsaturated fats, liquid at room temperature, are found in olive oil, canola oil, flaxseed oil, Enova brand oil, and fish oils.

Fish oils provide powerful omega-3 fatty acids, which have anti-inflammatory properties and are essential for good cardiovascular health and mental clarity. Our bodies need an optimal ratio of omega-6 to omega-3 fatty acids, generally between 4:1 and 10:1 (omega-6 to omega-3). (Our diets are typically much higher in omega-6 than omega-3.) The omega-3 fatty acids found in salmon, mackerel, lake trout, herring, sardines, tuna, and some types of white fish are essential, meaning that your body cannot make them and they must come from your diet. Unless you eat fish at least three times a week, you're not getting enough omega-3s.

Everyone should have a bottle of high-lignan flaxseed oil and/or fish oil in the refrigerator. Flaxseed oil is high in omega-3 and some omega-6 fatty acids, much like fish oil. A tablespoon or two a day—one in the morning and one in the evening—is all you need, and it can go into a post-workout recovery shake or on top of oatmeal.

Blended oils such as Udo's Choice Blend are another good option. Don't sacrifice the health benefits of these oils just because you can't stomach them in liquid form. Simply take them as pills. As with any supplement, check with your physician before taking the product.

PERFORMANCE POINTS:

● "Good" fats are vital for a healthy lifestyle. Examples include fish, olive oil, and nuts. Choose fats that provide nutritional value, not just empty calories.

- Avoid trans fats and examine labels carefully.

- Consider adding supplements such as flaxseed oil to your diet if you do not get the omega-3 you need from food.

ENDURANCE NUTRITION STRATEGY #4: EAT EARLY, OFTEN, AND BALANCED

Now that we've discussed the three main components of your meals, I want you to forget what you've been told about eating three square meals a day and avoiding between-meal snacks. If you want to control your blood sugar level (to improve concentration and regulate your appetite) and build lean body mass, you must eat six small to medium-size meals or snacks a day. That means you need to eat, on average, every 3 hours. Think of yourself as "grazing" throughout the day, instead of sitting for three big meals.

Remember this formula: "3 for 3." Eat all three nutrients every 3 hours for optimal energy and body composition.

Your metabolism is like a fire. It is in constant need of fuel. If you let it go for a long time without adding logs, the fire smolders and dies. Each time you eat (or add fuel) to the fire, it cranks up your metabolism and burns more calories to digest the food. You have an efficient, hot, burning metabolism.

As an endurance athlete, you've created this hot fire. If you don't continually toss more "wood" on it, it's going to turn to your valuable lean muscle mass and smolder. I recommend that everyone eat frequently, but it's especially important for endurance athletes, for whom a constant fuel supply is vital.

If we don't eat often, the most readily available substance for the body to consume is muscle. That's contrary to the popular belief that the first thing the body eats away is fat. The body is actually remarkably resistant to fat loss and will turn to its lean muscle mass first, keeping stored fat in reserve as long as possible.

Many endurance athletes try to stay thin by not eating. In fact, many people turn to endurance sports because they see them as a means to lose weight. They deprive their bodies of nutrients and, while they might look healthy, their bodies may be really out of balance.

When your body is not properly nourished, it begins a slippery slide of hormonal imbalance, a decrease in energy, and an inability to recovery efficiently. It begins to eat away at your muscle for energy. As an endurance athlete, you are eating to perform. You need to be in a constant fueled-up state to meet your energy needs. You want to feel great

BETWEEN-MEAL SNACKS

The key to eating six times a day is planning. Keep snacks in a desk drawer at work, in the car, in a diaper bag, briefcase, or backpack—wherever you need them to ensure that you'll never have to go more than 3 hours without at least a snack. Be sure to keep plenty of bottled water handy in these locations as well. You won't get hungry, and you won't have to spend time and money searching for the first available snack, which likely won't be a healthy option.

Here's a list of easy-to-assemble snacks that we recommend to our clients who train at the Athletes' Performance Institutes:

1 apple with 2 teaspoons peanut butter

1 pear with ½ cup low-fat, low-sugar yogurt

1 banana with 1 teaspoon peanut butter

1 cup low-fat, low-sugar yogurt mixed with ½ cup Kashi Go Lean cereal, and ⅛ cup almond slivers

1 cup low-fat, low-sugar frozen yogurt with ¼ cup fruit and ¼ cup nuts

1 can of tuna or chicken with a handful of whole wheat crackers

½ cup 1% cottage cheese with ¼ cup fruit

¼ cup almonds with ½ cup fruit

¼ cup peanuts with ½ cup fruit

½ peanut butter sandwich with 8 ounces 1% or fat-free milk

1 EAS Myoplex shake

1 EAS bar, such as Myoplex Lite, or a Clif bar, such as Clif Builder. PowerBar Triple Threat, and Luna are also good options.

The challenge with meal-replacement bars is to find something that tastes good and is also good for you. Look at the label carefully. Your goal is to find something with 15 to 30 grams of protein. It should have twice the amount of carbs when you're training (30 to 60 grams), and a few grams of fat. Be on the lookout for bars that contain high-fructose corn syrup—you'll want to avoid those. When choosing a bar for a snack, your eyes should head straight for the fiber line on the label. Try to find a bar with at least 3 grams of fiber. If it has 3 grams of fiber, go for it!

The ratio of protein to carbs depends on your activity level. If you're sitting in the office, go with a ratio of 1 gram of protein to 1 gram of carbs (1:1). If you're consuming a bar before or after training, go with 1 gram of protein to 2 to 3 grams of carbs (1: 2–3). If it's a heavy day of training, go with a 1:3 ratio. If your bar is too high in protein, simply add a fruit to that snack to bump up the carb content.

during your training, recover quickly from your sessions, and perform optimally.

The last thing you want to do is lose the lean mass you've worked so hard to achieve and put your body at a greater risk for injury. Lean mass produces power, stabilizes joints, promotes movement, and is critical for optimal performance.

The six "meals" are not going to be long, sit-down affairs. (We eat to live, not live to eat, right?) Three of them could be a combination of energy-rich, post-workout recovery shakes, a piece of fruit, a meal replacement bar, or a handful of nuts.

You could have three moderate-size meals and three small snacks, or you could have six meals of equal size. Your six "meals" will include snacks (mini-meals) and your recovery shake(s). Just remember to make sure that you account for all three nutrients (carbs, protein, and fat) every 3 hours.

Building the Perfect Meal

There should be a balance between carbs, proteins, and good fats in each of your meals. These meals should start early—as soon as you get up. One nutrition cliché that *is* true is that breakfast is the most important meal of the day. Your body has been in a fasted state since you went to bed, so it's important that you "break the fast" not long after rising and keep your body fueled all day long. I can't think of an easier, healthier breakfast than a cup of old-fashioned Quaker Oats and milk.

I'd rather you eat *anything* for breakfast than skip the meal. When I coached college athletes, I had such difficulty getting them to eat breakfast that I all but begged them to eat leftover pizza instead of going hungry. That's how important breakfast is. Even if you work out early in the morning, you need to fuel up before training. Research suggests that those who are fueled before runs or training sessions can go harder and longer.

As you build meals through the rest of your day, remember the three nutrients and judge your meals with your visual cues. With a little practice, all you will have to do is look at the plate, and you'll know whether it is going to fuel you optimally.

Typically, your plate should consist mostly of colorful vegetables. There should be a piece of meat or fish the size of a deck of cards and, if you like, a fist-size portion of brown rice or whole wheat pasta. (If this meal follows a training session or race, two fists is appropriate.) There also should be some "good" fat in the form of, say, salmon or olive oil.

I recommend that you "eat a rainbow often," which not only refers to the bright colors of fiber-rich fruits and vegetables that should be part of every meal but also reminds you to eat six small meals and snacks a day.

MEAL ASSEMBLY

These days it's difficult for anyone, especially endurance athletes, to find time to plan, prepare, and enjoy full-blown meals. That's why I find it valuable to "assemble" meals rather than cook or prepare them. (Remember, we're eating to live, not living to eat.)

Prepare for your week on Sunday by grilling a large quantity of chicken, fish, and lean red meat. Cut it into individual servings. Steam vegetables and slice tomatoes. Cook plenty of good carbs, such as sweet potatoes, brown rice, couscous, and whole wheat pasta. Grab some prepackaged salad mixes and place everything into single-serving containers. That way, you'll have plenty of food for the week ahead.

Another easy strategy is to purchase precooked rotisserie chickens, which are available for about $6 apiece at warehouse shopping centers. Peel off the skin, pat away the excess oil, cut up the bird, and you'll have enough meat for two to four single meals.

Not only will you have meals to get you through much of the workweek, but you also can put a small cooler in the car for those weekend days when you're out training or running errands. You'll find that the meal assembly process saves time and money and that it requires minimal effort to create a high-performance nutrition plan that's adaptable to any lifestyle.

MEAL PLAN FOR FEMALE ATHLETES

BREAKFAST	SNACK	LUNCH	SNACK	DINNER	SNACK
2 grains	1 supplement	2 grains	1 supplement	2 grains	1 fruit or vegetable
1 protein	OR	1 protein	OR	1 protein	and
1 fruit	1 grain or fruit and	1 fat	1 grain or fruit and	1 fat	1 protein or fat
1 fat	1 protein	1 fruit or vegetable	1 protein or fat	3 vegetable	OR
					1 supplement

MEAL PLAN FOR MALE ATHLETES

BREAKFAST	SNACK	LUNCH	SNACK	DINNER	SNACK
3 grains	1 supplement	3 grains	1 supplement	3 grains	2 fruits or vegetables
1 protein	OR	2 proteins	OR	2 proteins	and
1 fruit	2 grains or fruits and	1 fat	2 grains or fruits and	1 fat	1 protein or fat
1 fat	1 protein	1 fruit or vegetable	1 protein or fat	3 vegetables	OR
					1 supplement

HEALTHFUL MEAL COMPONENTS

The tables below will help you create healthful meals custom-tailored to your nutritional needs. These are just a starting point; keep in mind that the more active you are, the more carbs you will need. Make sure you get your meal or snack within 30 minutes after your workout!

GRAINS	PROTEIN		
	MEAT/EGG	DAIRY	VEGETARIAN
1 slice bread (whole wheat optimal)	4 oz turkey	½ c 1% cottage cheese	½ c tofu
½ bagel (whole wheat optimal)	4 oz skinless chicken	8 oz fat-free or 1% milk	½ c cooked beans
½ English muffin	4 oz lean roast beef	6 oz low-sugar, fat-free yogurt	½ c soy milk
1 whole wheat tortilla (6" size)	4 oz 96% lean ground beef		
1 c high fiber cereal (such as Kashi)	4 oz lean red meat		
½ c cooked oatmeal	4 oz tuna		
½ c brown rice	4 oz salmon or other fish		
½ c cooked pasta (whole wheat optimal)	2 eggs		
½ c cooked whole wheat couscous	4 egg whites		
1 medium baked sweet potato			
1 medium baked potato			

FRUITS	VEGETABLES	FATS	SUPPLEMENTS*
1 apple	½ c asparagus	1 Tbsp olive oil	EAS Myoplex Lite
1 banana	½ c bell pepper	1 Tbsp flaxseed oil (do not cook with this)	Myoplex Lite RTD
1 c berries (fresh or frozen)	½ c carrots	½ avocado	*Athletes' Performance Institutes exclusively use EAS products for athlete supplementation because of their banned-substance-free certification from NSF, a nonprofit, nongovernmental organization, and our strong belief in the efficacy of the products.
1 grapefruit	½ c green beans	¼ c peanuts, walnuts, or almonds	
1 orange	½ c mushrooms	¼ c low-fat cheese	
1 peach	1 c spinach (raw or frozen)	1 slice low fat cheese	
1 nectarine	1 c romaine lettuce	2 Tbsp low fat dressing	
1½ c grapes	½ c celery	1 Tbsp regular dressing	
21 cherries	½ c cooked or raw vegetables	1 tsp butter	
8 strawberries	1 c raw leafy vegetables	1 Tbsp peanut butter	
½ c to ¾ c 100% fruit juice		1 Tbsp Enova oil	
½ c cooked or canned fruit (canned in its own juice)		1 Tbsp fish oil	

PERFORMANCE POINTS:

● Think "3 for 3." Eat a combination of carbs, proteins, and fats every 3 hours.

● Allowing your body to go long periods without eating contributes to low energy levels, subpar performance, and breakdown.

● Following a consistent pattern of fueling throughout the day contributes to increased energy and lean mass.

ENDURANCE NUTRITION STRATEGY #5: STAY HYDRATED

If you take a dry sponge, dip it in a bucket of water, and pull it right out, it remains dry. Maybe it absorbed a little water, but nothing substantial. When it comes to hydration, your muscle cells are like that sponge. If you wait to hydrate immediately before or during a training session, while you're sweating, it will be tough to hydrate your body's "sponge" adequately.

If you hydrate over the course of the day, you retain the moisture in your body's sponge all day long. This is important for everyone, but especially for endurance athletes. Even minor dehydration impairs concentration, coordination, and reaction time. It reduces stamina and compromises the body's ability to resist disease.

Dehydration of just 3 percent can cause a 10 percent loss of strength and an 8 percent loss of speed. There's no simpler way to maintain—and improve—performance than by staying properly hydrated. In fact, just drinking enough water before, during, and after exercise can increase performance by up to 25 percent. A good rule of thumb is to drink ½ to 1 ounce of water per pound of body weight per day to maintain hydration.

When you think of hydration, divide it into hydration for "everyday" and hydration for "performance." To maintain proper hydration during the day, noncaloric beverages such as water or green tea are the best things to be drinking.

Now when you start considering hydration for performance, think of hydration as a means of replacing what you are losing. If your event or training session lasts longer than an hour, or if you are in an extreme environment with heat and humidity, sports drinks that have a glucose content of 6 to 10 percent and that contain sodium and potassium are effective. Gatorade, Cytomax, EAS Endurathon, and Amino Vital Endurance are good examples.

Sodium balance is important for endurance athletes; however, it is really important to those who are "salty sweaters," people who lose more sodium in their sweat and tend to cramp and become fatigued quicker. If you find that you are a salty sweater (for example, you often have a white film on your clothing and a salty layer on your skin) you may need a carbohydrate electrolyte beverage with a higher amount of sodium, such as Gatorade Endurance, EAS Endurathon, or Amino Vital Endurance.

Gatorade has been a pioneer in research relating to hydration and performance. At the Athletes' Performance Institutes, we are excited to partner with Gatorade to perform research on some of our athletes. What we have found is that athletes were losing sodium through their intense training, validating the use of an electrolyte replacement beverage during their sessions.

Don't assume that sports drinks are an adequate substitute for water in everyday life. Sports drinks are designed to enhance sport performance. They are not meant to be consumed throughout the day while you're sitting at your desk or watching television. Many of them are loaded with high-glycemic carbohydrates that elevate blood sugar and ultimately contribute to body fat if not needed to fuel activity. But when you are competing and training for prolonged, intense periods, sports drinks are critical for performance.

I'm sure you know the pitfalls of caffeine, alcohol, and soda. Targeted caffeine use does have benefits for endurance athletes (see "Targeted Caffeine Use" on page 99), but caffeine should not be used as a daily energy source, the way millions of Americans use it. By following the Core Performance Endurance workout and nutrition program, you won't need to rely on stimulants just to get through the day.

Coffee—black coffee, not creamy, sugary coffee drinks—has antioxidant properties and when consumed in moderation can help meet your antioxidant needs. For better or for worse, coffee often is the highest source of antioxidants for Americans. Antioxidants *should* come from a variety of healthful fruits and vegetables and from a variety of other healthful drinks (in addition to coffee) such as green, white, or black tea. All of these teas have different, protective antioxidant properties.

Soda is loaded with sugar or with fat-producing high-fructose corn syrup. Did you know that there are roughly 15 spoonfuls of sugar in just one 12-ounce can of soda? Diet soda is better, but it does not offer the same benefits as water.

I also recommend limiting alcohol intake to an occasional glass of red wine, which, according to several studies, reduces the risk of multiple disease profiles.

I know it's tough to alter one's liquid intake, since it's such an ingrained part of day-to-day life. But there's no easier way to maintain consistent energy levels, regulate appetite, boost performance in sports, and improve overall health than to substitute water for whatever kind of soda, caffeinated beverage, or alcoholic drink dominates your life.

My coauthor, Pete Williams, used to drink about six diet sodas a day. He'd put away even more on days when he ate out, not realizing how often the server refilled his glass. Now, he follows what he calls the "Biblical Beverage Plan," drinking nothing but water, including water mixed with post-workout recovery mixes, and an occasional glass of wine. He feels better, gets more benefit from his workouts, has healthier teeth, and no longer relies on caffeine to get through the day. He even saves money.

Pete eats plenty of fruit, so he's getting the benefits of juice—plus all of the fiber and other nutrients that would have been squeezed out during juicing. Like anyone, he'll need some Amino Vital or Gatorade if he embarks on some serious endurance training. Other than that, he doesn't need anything other than what's been available since the beginning of time to stay properly hydrated.

PERFORMANCE POINTS:

● Drink ½ to 1 ounce of water per pound of body weight per day to maintain hydration.

● Think before you drink. Don't hydrate with high-sugar beverages such as soda and fruit drinks.

● Use sports drinks for improving performance. If your training is longer than an hour or if it takes place in intense heat, use a carbohydrate-electrolyte or a carbohydrate+electrolyte+protein drink to enhance your performance.

CHAPTER 7 SUMMARY: Endurance training creates heavy nutritional demands, but many endurance athletes often fail to fuel their bodies properly. The key is to recognize that nutrition goes a long way toward determining performance and overall health. Even amid a hectic schedule, it's possible to eat for optimum health and performance. Good strategies include eating every 3 hours; finding a proper balance of carbs, proteins, and fats; and staying properly hydrated.

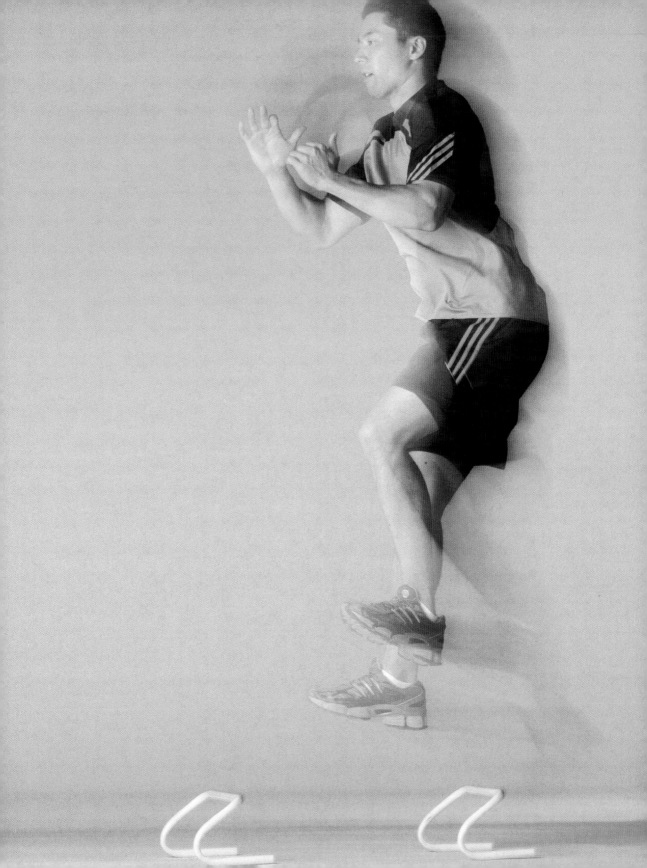

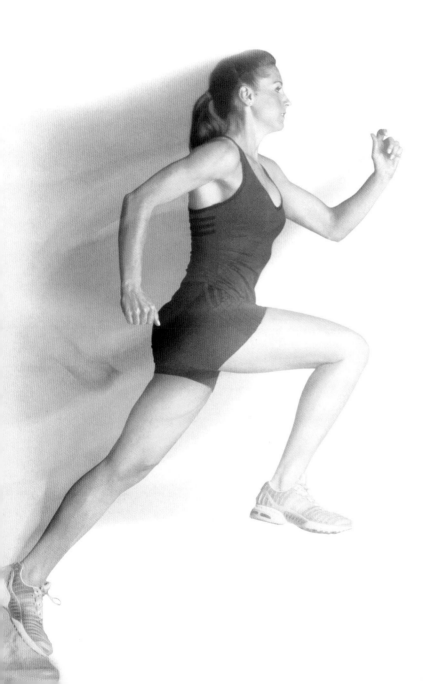

CHAPTER 8

TIMING IS EVERYTHING

With the five strategies discussed in the last chapter, you've set yourself up well for everyday nutrition. You're eating often—six times a day—and you've struck a balance between carbohydrates, protein, and good fats to maximize performance. You're also staying properly hydrated.

By planning out your "perfect day," you will be able to optimize nutrition for performance. The biggest barriers to effective nutrition are planning and implementation. If you can plot your perfect day and follow through, you're well on your way to success.

We're also going to take things a step further by adding some supplementation strategies that will contribute to performance. This falls into two categories—the way you eat and supplement on a normal training day and what you'll want to do before, during, and after competitions or intense training sessions.

When fueling and refueling for training sessions and competitions, think of three time periods: pre, during, and post. You never want your body to be deprived of key nutrients, especially when working out. It is important to fuel your body for each session, giving it the nutrients it needs during the workout and then refueling after the training session.

HOW TO EAT ON A NORMAL TRAINING DAY
Before Your Workout

Before your training session or run, hydrate and consume carbs and protein. An easy way to do this is to down a pre-workout "shooter," which is simply a watered-down glass of orange juice with a scoop of whey protein. Recent research has shown that the pre-workout "shooter" may produce an effect equal to a traditional post-workout recovery shake. The pre-workout shooter works its way into your bloodstream to give your muscle exactly what it needs at the earliest possible moment.

EAS makes a great product called Endurathon. One scoop of this mixed with 8 to 12 ounces of water, or a half bottle of Gatorade plus one scoop of whey, will help to fuel your run or training session.

During Your Workout

During your training sessions or runs, be sure to consider the intensity and the duration. You should start drinking early and at regular intervals in an attempt to replace water lost through sweating. Regardless of the intensity, make sure that you drink 4 to 6 gulps of fluid every 10 to 20 minutes.

If the session is more than 45 minutes or in intense heat, consume a carbohydrate-electrolyte or carbohydrate+electrolyte+protein drink. For performance benefits, you'll want to consume the equivalent of 30 to 60 grams of carbs per hour. This will ensure that you are properly fueled and feeling great during the session. You will find 30 grams of carbs in 16 ounces of Gatorade; 1 scoop of Amino Vital Endurance; one packet of Gu, Hammer Gel, or Clif Shot; 2 scoops of EAS Endurathon; or 1 packet of Cytomax.

After Your Workout

To refuel your body after a workout or run, consume a mixture of carbohydrates and protein immediately afterward. I recommend a post-workout recovery shake such as Myoplex or Myoplex Lite. Liquid forms of nutrition are designed to be digested and absorbed quickly. These prepackaged, convenient shakes contain an effective ratio of proteins, carbohydrates, and fat, and they are loaded with fiber, vitamins, and minerals.

I strongly recommend Myoplex products, made by EAS, one of my company's strategic partners. Could you get the same value in similar products from other manufacturers? Perhaps, though EAS is the only company to earn the "banned-substance-free" and "accuracy in labeling" certification.

Ideally, you should have a shake right after

the workout. At that point, your cells are wide open and screaming for nutrients, and by drinking one of these shakes, you expedite the recovery process and maximize lean-muscle growth.

By getting a mix of carbs and protein, you'll help repair muscle, replenish your fuel stores, and rehydrate your body. This also improves your postrace and post-workout stress hormone profile. After a race or intense training session, you have high levels of the stress hormone cortisol. Testosterone, which is found in men and women and plays an important role in immune function, is at a low level at this point.

With this nutritional intervention, we can raise the testosterone level and lower the cortisol level. The benefits go far beyond the short term. By addressing your nutritional needs within 10 minutes of training, you're jump-starting the recovery process.

PERFORMANCE POINTS:

● PRETRAINING: Consume a "shooter" with 15 to 30 grams of carbs and 5 to 10 grams of protein, along with 16 ounces of water.

● DURING THE WORKOUT: Consume 4 to 6 gulps of water or sports drink every 10 to 20 minutes.

● POST-WORKOUT: Consume protein (body weight in pounds ÷ 2.2 × 0.4) + carbohydrates (body weight in pounds ÷ 2.2 × 0.8). Though these formulas might look complex, all we're doing is taking your body weight in pounds and dividing it by

2.2 to convert to kilograms. From there, we're multiplying to get the number of grams needed.

Because everyone who reads this will be on a slightly different schedule, there's no one-size-fits-all routine I can offer. But if you remember the priorities—eating often and incorporating a pre-workout shooter and/or a post-workout recovery shake or meal—you can plan your day accordingly. (I'll even customize this to your exact schedule at our Web site, www.coreperformance.com/endurance, to remove any guesswork.)

Now that we've established this solid foundation for everyday eating and supplementation, let's take it a step further and examine what you need to do to get ready for a big training session or a longer endurance competition such as a 10-K, 10-miler, half-marathon, marathon, or triathlon.

HOW TO EAT BEFORE TRAINING AND COMPETITION

We can break down "event nutrition" into five categories:

1. The night before the race

2. Four hours before the race or 2 hours before the race

3. One hour before the race

4. Immediately before the race

5. Immediately after the race

PERFECT TIMING

**This table makes it easy to see what types of foods
you should eat when, and for which types of events.**

TYPES OF EVENTS	TIMING	CARBOHYDRATE/FOOD RECOMMENDATIONS	SAMPLE FOODS
Endurance events Intermediate distances Short-duration events	The night before	Higher-carb meal: 300 g carbs in meal and snack Moderate in fiber Easy on the fat Plenty of fluid	Pasta dishes Rice dishes Lean protein Cooked veggies Fruit
Endurance events Intermediate distances	3 to 4 hours prior	Carbs: 1.5 g per lb body weight Low-fat protein Low fat and fiber Plenty of fluids	Cereals, bread, crackers Milk Fruit, juices, jelly
Short-duration events Intermediate distances Endurance events Multiple events	2 hours prior	Carbs: 0.5 to 1 g per lb body weight Minimal, low-fat protein Low fat and low fiber	Cereals, bread, crackers Milk Fruit, juices, jelly
Short-duration events Intermediate-length events Endurance events Multiple events in one day	1 hour prior	Emphasize liquids Easy-to-digest carbs Avoid protein, fat, and fiber	Sports drinks Concentrated carb supplements Energy bars Tolerated fruits Water
Any event requiring carbohydrates and hydration	Immediately prior	Carbs	Sports drinks or Energy bars
Endurance events lasting longer than 45 minutes	During	30 to 60 g carbs per hour Carbohydrate+electrolyte or Carbohydrate+protein+electrolyte	Energy gel or Sports drinks or Energy bars

Any event	Immediately after, and meals within the 2-hour window of recovery	Carbs and whey/casein protein mix
		
		Use this formula: Protein (body weight ÷ 2.2 × 0.4) + carbohydrates (body weight ÷ 2.2 × 0.8)
			Immediately after:
			  Shakes
			  Energy bars
			  (EAS Myoplex Lite)
			  Sports drinks
			  Fruits
			Meals:
			  Pasta
			  Rice
			  Vegetables
			  Fruits
			  Lean meats

Sample Pre-Event Meals

The meals listed below might seem breakfastlike; indeed, they will be your first meal of the day. After all, most events start early in the morning. They are, however, more like quick fuel stops to prepare your body for competition.

We constructed these meals to provide significant fuel, but not so much that it's going to bog you down.

PRE-EVENT MEAL #1:

390 calories and 75 grams carbohydrates

2 slices of toast or 1 small bagel

1 large banana

1 tablespoon jelly

1 tablespoon peanut butter

Water

PRE-EVENT MEAL #2:

750 calories and 150 grams carbohydrates

2 slices of bread or 1 small bagel

1 cup yogurt with fruit

1 large banana

2 teaspoons peanut butter

2 tablespoons jelly

4 ounces 100% fruit juice

PRE-EVENT MEAL #3:

470 calories and 88 grams carbohydrates

Blend 1 cup vanilla yogurt, 4 to 6 peach halves, and 4 graham cracker squares or 1 cup of your favorite cereal.

PRE-EVENT MEAL #4:

895 calories and 147 grams carbohydrates

1 cup orange juice

¾ cup Grape-Nuts

1 large banana

1 cup fat-free milk

2 slices of toast with 1 tablespoon peanut butter and 2 tablespoons jelly

POST-EVENT OR POST-TRAINING

It is ideal to consume a shake, energy bar, and/or sports drink immediately following training or games. Do this before you do anything else. The food or supplement you choose should provide about 0.8 gram of carbohydrates per kilogram of body weight and 0.4 gram of protein per kilogram of body weight. Pick and choose again from the list below for optimal choices.

Carbohydrate need:

(Your body weight in pounds ÷ 2.2)

× 0.8 gram = _____

Protein need:

(Your body weight in pounds ÷ 2.2)

× 0.4 gram = _____

Mix and match the following foods to meet your carbohydrate needs. Except where noted, each food listed contains 30 grams of carbohydrates.

CEREALS AND STARCHES

Breads

Bagel, ½ whole

Cornbread, 1 square

Dinner rolls, 2

English muffin, 1 whole

Pita pocket, 1

Whole wheat bread, 2 slices

Cereals

Cold cereal, ¾ to 1 cup

Cooked cereal (oatmeal), 1 cup

Grape-Nuts, ⅓ cup

Shredded Wheat, ¾ cup

Grains

Graham crackers, 6 squares

Pancakes, 4-inch, 3

Pasta, cooked, 1 cup

Rice, cooked white or brown, ⅔ cup

Tortillas, corn or flour, 2

Waffle, 1 large

STARCHY VEGETABLES

Baked beans, cooked, ¾ cup

Black beans, cooked, ¾ cup

Corn, cooked, ¾ cup

Kidney beans, cooked, ¾ cup

Peas, cooked, 1 cup

Popcorn, no oil, 5 cups

Potato, baked, 1 medium

Sweet potato, baked, 4 ounces

Vegetables

Asparagus, boiled, 1 cup

Beans, green, boiled, 1 cup

Broccoli, boiled, 1 cup

Broccoli, raw, 2 cups

Carrots, cooked, ⅔ cup

Carrots, raw, 2

Fruits

Apple, 1½ medium

Applesauce, sweetened, ½ cup

Applesauce, unsweetened, 1 cup

Apricots, raw, 8 medium

Banana, 1 large

Blueberries, raw, 1½ cups

Cantaloupe, raw, 2 cups, cubed

Fruit salad, 1 cup

Grapefruit, 1 large

Grapes, small, 1 cup

Honeydew, ¼ melon

Kiwifruits, 3 medium

Mango, 1 medium

Oranges, 2 medium

Nectarines, 2

Peaches, 2

Plums, 3 medium

Raisins, ⅓ cup (about 3 tablespoons)

Fruit and Vegetable Juices

Apple juice, 8 ounces

Carrot juice, 10 ounces

Cranberry juice cocktail, 8 ounce

Grape juice, 6 ounces

Grapefruit or orange juice, 8 ounces

CARB LOADING, ANYONE?

These days, the notion of carb loading is viewed as old school, even outdated. But if your event is going to last longer than 90 minutes, you might benefit from carb loading. The idea is to give your muscles and liver a little extra fuel, sort of like topping off the tank. Don't stress over carb loading; just make some simple adjustments to your diet to optimize your fuel stores. Here are some steps to perfect your carb loading:

- Make sure to meet your carb needs every day. Carb loading the day before the race isn't going to make up for inadequate carb intake over the duration of your training cycle. Make sure to match your carb intake with your intensity level (2 to 5 grams of carbs per pound of body weight per day), and be sure to get the proper amount of carbs in your recovery meal or snack.

- Taper the training, but don't taper the carbs. As you begin to taper your training before an event, do not cut back on your carb intake. The decrease in activity will decrease your fuel needs; therefore, the extra carbs that you are eating will be used to supercompensate your fuel stores.

- Go big at lunch, not dinner, the day before the race. Consume your heavier-carb meal at lunch the day before the race. Follow it with a normal dinner and an evening snack. This allows the carbs from the meal to be digested and shuttled to your fuel stores.

Pineapple juice, 8 ounces

Vegetable juice cocktail, 24 ounces

SWEETS

Chocolate milk, 8 ounces

Granola bar, 1

Honey, 2 tablespoons

Jam, 2 tablespoons

Jelly, 2 tablespoons

Syrup, 2 tablespoons

MILK/YOGURT

Varying carbohydrate content

Milk, fat-free or 2%, 8 ounces (12 g carbs)

Yogurt, fat-free, 8 ounces (15 g carbs)

Yogurt, fat-free with fruit, 8 ounces (30 to 45 g carbs)

CARB CONTENT OF COMMON SPORTS NUTRITION SUPPLEMENTS

PowerBar: 40 grams

Gatorade, 16 ounces: 28 grams

Cytomax, 1 scoop: 20 grams

Clif Shot: 46 grams

Clif Bar: 51 grams

Myoplex Lite Bar: 28 grams

Myoplex Deluxe Bar: 36 grams

Myoplex Lite/Original shake: 20 grams

RACE DAY SPECIFICS
Before Competition

You need fuel to compete. During long events, or when you haven't eaten in some time, blood glucose levels fall, zapping your energy, concentration, and mood. Low blood sugar during a long training session or race can hinder performance dramatically.

The pre-event meal serves two purposes. It prevents you from feeling hungry and provides adequate glucose to your muscles, blood, and liver. Below are suggestions for what to eat and when for your pre-event meal.

FOOD CHOICES 2 TO 4 HOURS BEFORE AN EVENT

Your pre-event meal should be high in carbohydrates, though not exclusively carbs. Carbs digest and absorb quickly into the bloodstream, enabling you to work out without the proverbial brick of food sitting in the stomach. An empty stomach is less prone to indigestion and nausea.

EVENT PLANNING AT A GLANCE

EVENTS LASTING 60 MINUTES OR LESS

PRE-EVENT: This is a short race. Make sure to eat something with carbs and a little protein and hydrate with about 16 to 20 ounces of fluid. More important, make sure to eat sensibly in the days leading up to the race and make sure that you recover after your training sessions. Examples: Toast with peanut butter, one-half or an entire energy bar, a 16-ounce sports drink.

DURING: Grab water or a sports drink every 10 to 15 minutes.

POST-EVENT: Consume a mixture of carbs and protein as quickly as possible after the race. An energy bar or ready-to-drink product is the easiest option.

EVENTS LASTING MORE THAN 60 MINUTES

PRE-EVENT: Drink 17 to 20 ounces of water 2 hours before the race. Consume 7 to 10 ounces of a sports drink 10 to 20 minutes before the race. Consume 1 to 2 carbs per pound of body weight 2 to 4 hours before the race.

DURING: Consume 30 to 60 grams of carbs per hour from liquid, solid, or semi-solid sources. Drink 7 to 10 ounces of fluid every 10 to 15 minutes. If the event is longer than a 90-minute duration, choose a carbohydrate+electrolyte+protein or amino acid beverage.

POST-EVENT: Consume 0.8 gram of carbs per kilogram of body weight plus 0.4 gram of protein per kilogram of body weight immediately after the race, followed by another meal 60 to 90 minutes later. Drink 16 ounces of sports drink for each pound lost.

Choose from these foods:

Grains—rice, breads, bagels, pasta, and cereal

Fruits—apples, oranges, and bananas

Other plant sources—potatoes, corn or peas, peanut butter

Animal sources—low-fat milk, low-fat yogurt, turkey, chicken breast, lean red meat, or low-fat cheese

Note: Beware of foods that are high in fat and fiber in these pre-event meals. Foods high in fiber can cause unexpected pit stops, and high-fat foods can cause nausea or vomiting during an event.

FOOD CHOICES 1 HOUR BEFORE AN EVENT OR RUN

Fruit and vegetable juices

Fresh fruit

Breads, bagels, low-fat yogurt, raisins

High-carb beverages (such as your favorite sports drink)

One serving commercial carbohydrate-electrolyte beverage

Consuming something—anything—is better than nothing before an event. Eating in the hour before a run can boost performance by 12.5 percent, according to several studies. At the very least, try to put away between 15 and 75 grams of carbs in the hour before any event. Here are some additional ideas for snacks that will help to give you the fuel you need:

Gatorade, 8 ounces: 15 grams

PowerBar Gel, 1.4 ounces: 28 grams

Gu, 1.1 ounces: 25 grams

Raisins, 1 ounce (about 2 tablespoons): 23 grams

Banana, small: 21 grams

PowerBar: 45 grams

Honey Nut Cheerios, without milk, ¾ cup (1 ounce): 23 grams

Bagel, Lender's 2-ounce: 30 grams

Bagel, typical New York: 40+ grams

Raisin bread, 1 slice: 16 grams

Nabisco Fig Newton, 1 cookie: 11 grams

Barnum's Animal Crackers, 12 cookies: 23 grams

Apple, 2¾-inch diameter: 15 grams

PRACTICE BEFORE PERFORMANCE

Be sure to practice with snacks during training sessions to determine your tolerance for different foods. Never try an unfamiliar product before or during competition. Experiment with different snacks and then establish a routine of whatever works for you. Be sure to record your choices in a training diary. On the day of the event, the prerace meal will be one less item to worry about. New foods and drinks may send you running for the Porta Potti! The final thing to think about prerace is hydration. You don't want to be like that dry sponge before a competition, so it's important to be well-hydrated with 8 to 16 ounces of water or sports drink.

During Competition

As we discussed earlier, it is crucial to stay hydrated and fueled during activity to ensure optimal performance. You want to maintain your fuel stores during competition so that you can perform at a higher level throughout the race but also to maintain energy reserves for a strong finish. After all, endurance events are wars of attrition. Think of glycogen stores as your critical energy reserve. You don't want to tap into them until you absolutely have to, when you need that extra "kick" to finish the race.

For races under 1 hour, such as 5-Ks and 10-Ks, you need not worry about replenishing glycogen stores until after the race. During events, athletes should start drinking early and at regular intervals in an attempt to replace all the water lost through sweat-

WATER INTOXICATION

It's difficult to overstate the importance of proper hydration for enhancing performance and health. A lack of water is dangerous. In extreme instances, athletes have suffered heat stroke and even died from dehydration.

But it's also possible to go overboard with hydration. *Hyponatremia,* also known as "water intoxication," is a potentially fatal condition experienced by endurance athletes who overhydrate with water.

This condition is brought on by extremely low blood sodium levels and triggers symptoms from nausea and muscle cramps to coma and even death. A runner died from the condition following the 2002 Boston Marathon, and another spent 4 days in a coma following a marathon in Jamaica.

The problem happens when there's too much water and not enough electrolytes (potassium, sodium, and chloride) flowing through the body. Water keeps coming in, but because of a lack of electrolytes, the blood sodium level is low, which throws off your heartbeat and response systems.

People tend to think that water is a better choice than sports drinks, since it has no calories. This is certainly true in everyday life. But when competing in an event or a training session of extreme exertion, it's important to hydrate with products that can replenish electrolytes. Good choices include Gatorade and Amino Vital Endurance Formula, or you can take products such as GatorLytes, Gu, or Hammer Gel with water.

ing. Drink an average of 1 cup (8 ounces) every 10 to 15 minutes.

If your event is longer than 60 minutes or if it is very intense, a sports drink can be substituted for water, and it will help replenish electrolytes. With longer races, you'll also want to consume 30 to 60 grams of carbs per hour. Your sports drink should provide 30 to 60 grams of carbs per hour. You could also get your carbs from energy bars or packet products. If you go that route, though, make sure you drink enough water as well.

You'll find 30 grams of carbs—enough to keep you going—in 16 ounces of Gatorade, one scoop of Amino Vital Endurance, one packet of Gu, Hammer Gel, or Clif Shot, or one packet of Cytomax.

Whatever your strategy, be sure to try it out long before the race, during one of your longer training sessions. That way, it will become an ingrained part of your routine. You never want to consume something new on the day of the race, since it could hinder performance.

After Competition

The race is done. You have accomplished a goal, but your body still is screaming for nutrients. I recommend that you refuel, rehydrate, and *then* celebrate. The recovery process starts the second you cross the finish line—or at least it should.

The sooner you consume nutrients, the better. You are compromising recovery by waiting even a half-hour to eat. Your post-race supplement should be just like your post-workout supplement. Eat mostly carbs but also some protein.

At the very least, eat a banana or drink a Gatorade or 16 ounces of low-fat chocolate milk. You'd get even more of a benefit from an EAS Myoplex shake. If you want to embark on world-class recovery, take the shake along with a multivitamin or antioxidant, plus a couple of fish oil capsules. You should drink 2 cups (16 ounces) for every pound lost during exercise. You might not notice a difference in how you feel, but over the long haul, you'll recover faster and perform better.

THE SCOOP ON SUPPLEMENTS

If you're a serious endurance athlete, you've probably heard a lot about supplementation, either from your friends or from reading or both. (We touched on amino acids in Chapter 7.) Some supplements can play an important role in building muscle before an event, and during an event, they can give you increased energy and stamina to propel you toward a strong finish. But not all supplements are created equal. This section will help you determine which supplement to use and when.

Putting Supplements in Their Place

Vitamins are catalysts that regulate reactions within your body. You must get vitamins from your diet because your body cannot make them. Nutritional deficiencies develop over the course of months or years of inadequate intake. My motto is "food first, supplement second!" There is no pill that can completely replicate the delicate balance of vitamins, minerals, and phytochemicals that occur naturally in food. But there is no denying that you need vitamins for your body to function at an optimal level; therefore, if you are not getting everything you need from food, supplements can be a part of your perfect day.

Keep in mind that when it comes down to

SIMPLE GUIDE TO SUPPLEMENTS

SUPPLEMENT	CATEGORY	FUNCTION
Antioxidants (Vitamins C and E)	Health Immune system function and recovery	Vitamins C and E work together to guard against oxidative stress. Exercise causes additional oxidative stress, so vitamins C and E may help to protect your immune system and speed recovery.
Branched chain amino acids (BCAAs)	Immune function and recovery	BCAAs may provide a fuel source for prolonged exercise, could help to delay fatigue, and may enhance immunity.
Caffeine	Stimulant	Stimulates the central nervous system, leading to a hightened sense of awareness and a decreased perception of effort. May spare muscle glycogen.
Calcium	Bone health	Many endurance runners restrict calories, and many female runners restrict dairy. Calcium deficiency can cause serious negative outcomes for bone health.
Carbohydrates	Fuel and recovery	Carbs provide fuel to the muscles and brain before, during, and after exercise. After exercise, carbs refuel the muscle and spike insulin, which brings the body's stress hormones down and back into balance.

performance, there is very little evidence to prove that extreme supplementation will enhance performance. There is, however, a lot of evolving research suggesting that certain supplements (antioxidants and glutamine) in monitored doses may help with recovery. The table below is a good starting point. Don't forget to talk to your physician before adding any supplements to your diet.

Glutamine: The Secret Weapon

One of the most effective supplements you can add to your training regimen is glutamine, a nonessential amino acid that plays an important role in keeping muscles functioning normally.

"Nonessential" means that the body can produce its own supply of glutamine if you

SAFETY/EFFICACY	AMOUNT	TIMING
Keep your levels of vitamins C and E in check. Just because they may be good doesn't mean you need to go crazy. Tolerable Upper Daily Limits: Vitamin C: 2,000 mg Vitamin E: 1,000 mg	Vitamin C: 250 to 500 mg Vitamin E: 250 to 500 mg	After exercise
Seem to be safe. Promising studies are related to immune system support.	5 to 20 g, in divided doses, seems to be safe	Before, during, and after exercise
Considered safe, but may cause an increase in blood pressure, heart rate, GI distress, and can cause withdrawal symptoms (headache) for chronic users. Effective CNS stimulant.	2.5 to 6 mg/kg body weight	60 min prior to event
Calcium supplements can help make up any dietary deficiencies. Those who train for 90 minutes in the heat also have greater needs. Do not exceed 2,500 mg per day.	If a dietary deficiency exists, supplement 1 or 2 times per day with a product that contains calcium and vitamin D.	Daily, between meals
Research suggests that high-glycemic carbs cause a quick and strong insulin response. This response helps the body to recovery quickly and efficiently. No safety issues with high-GI carbs after workouts!	Your fuel needs depend on your training load. During intense training sessions or competitions, consume 30 to 60 g carbs per hour. After training sessions and runs, consume 0.8 g/kg body weight.	Consume low-glycemic carbs before workouts and during the day. Consume high-glycemic carbs during and after training.

(continued)

SIMPLE GUIDE TO SUPPLEMENTS (CONTINUED)

SUPPLEMENT	CATEGORY	FUNCTION
Essential fatty acids	Inflammation control	When the body has enough omega-3 fatty acid, there is a decrease in blood clotting and inflammatory responses in the body. Serious deficiencies can lead to skin disorders, diarrhea, and anemia.
Glutamine	Immune function and recovery	Glutamine may decrease after strenuous exercise. Supplemental glutamine may help decrease exercise-induced stress.
Leucine	Recovery	Adding leucine to a carbohydrate-protein mixture has been shown to enhance recovery and muscle repair.
Multivitamin	Health	There is no scientific evidence that everyone should consume a multivitamin; however, many respected scientists recommend it to cover any deficiencies. If you are restricting calorie intake and know that your diet is lacking, a multivitamin is recommended.
Whey /casein protein	Immune function and recovery	Whey and casein are both milk proteins. Whey is quickly digested and well absorbed. It also has other immune and antioxidant properties. Casein is digested slower and provides prolonged nutrients for recovery.

are not taking it in through foods such as poultry and fish. In addition to its muscular benefits, glutamine is used by white blood cells and contributes to immune system function. It's especially beneficial for people whose immune systems have been compromised, such as those suffering from serious burns, cancer, and even AIDS.

Most people produce enough glutamine.

Then again, most people don't undergo serious endurance training that places a huge demand on the immune system and makes you more susceptible to illness.

As with everything else in the Core Performance Endurance program, we want to be proactive about nutrition. So make it a point to add glutamine to your nutritional plan. You'll find it in EAS Myoplex powders and

SAFETY/EFFICACY	AMOUNT	TIMING
Safe for healthy individuals in doses that do not exceed 3 g daily. Anything over 3 g per day should be supervised by a physician. Those who are on any medications, especially anticoagulants, should check with their doctor before beginning supplementation.	1 to 3 g of EPA/DHA or fish oil 1 to 2 Tbsp of flaxseed oil 1 Tbsp/50 lb of body weight for essential fatty acid blends	Anytime during the day. Take with meals in divided doses. Great as a part of a post-workout shake.
No known adverse effects when taken in recommended dose. Research is mixed and inconclusive.	5 to 20 g, in divided doses	Pre-, during, and/or post-workout
More and more research is coming out on this topic, and prelimnary results look promising enough to add this to your post-workout shake.	1 tsp or 3 g total	Post-workout recovery shake— mixed with protein and carbohydrates
Research and recommendations are mixed on the topic of multivitamins. Effective to reverse nutrient deficiencies. As long as the multivitamin does not cause you to go over your daily needs, there should be no harm.	Avoid megadosing. Megadosing the fat-soluble vitamins (A, D, E, K) may be particularly dangerous because these are stored in the fat and may build up to toxic levels.	Daily
Protein supplements are quick and easy ways to get protein during the day and after activity. There is nothing unsafe about additional protein; just make sure not to go well over your recommended daily intake.	Protein supplements should make up part of your daily protein intake of up to 0.8 g/lb of body weight. Pre: 5 to 15 g During: 5 to 15 g Post: 0.4 g/kg body weight	Before, during, and after exercise

other EAS products. You can get a tub of glutamine powder and add it to shakes and drinks. It's valuable to consume pre- or post-workout. Make it a point to get between 10 and 12 grams of glutamine each day.

Targeted Caffeine Use

You don't want caffeine to become a daily part of your lifestyle or even a regular part of your training. But when used on occasion, it's a proven training aid for endurance athletes.

It's most effective for longer-duration workouts, especially on days when you feel sluggish. Caffeine stimulates the central nervous system, causes the body to use fat as fuel more effectively, and preserves muscle glycogen. You'll feel more energetic, and your perceived rate of exertion will be lower.

Our research at the Athletes' Performance Institutes has found that caffeine significantly improves peak power outputs, especially when athletes need a special push. Generally speaking, the recommended dose is about 5 milligrams per kilogram of body weight (divide your weight by 2.2 to translate pounds into kilograms). For example, a 150-pound athlete would need 300 to 350 milligrams of caffeine to experience performance-enhancing benefits. An easy way to do this would be to use 1.5 scoops of Catapult. It's one of my favorite caffeine products, produced by EAS, one of my company's sponsors.

Don't employ this targeted caffeine strategy for the first time before a big event. Try it before a training session first. Check with your doctor before using caffeine if you have high blood pressure or a heart condition.

Again, caffeine is not something you want to use on a regular basis. You'll develop a tolerance for it and minimize its effectiveness. That could inspire you to take heavier doses, leading to dependency and other complications. But when used sparingly, it can be a valuable boost to performance.

CHAPTER 8 SUMMARY: Timing of meals and snacks has a significant effect on an endurance athlete's performance. Consuming different foods at specific points before, during, and after an event or strenuous training session can help you optimize your performance and ease recovery. In addition to maintaining a healthy diet for day-to-day living, successful endurance performance depends on proper supplementation, both on a daily basis and through a targeted strategy for pre-event, during-event, and post-event consumption. These strategies include post-workout recovery mixes, glutamine, and targeted caffeine use.

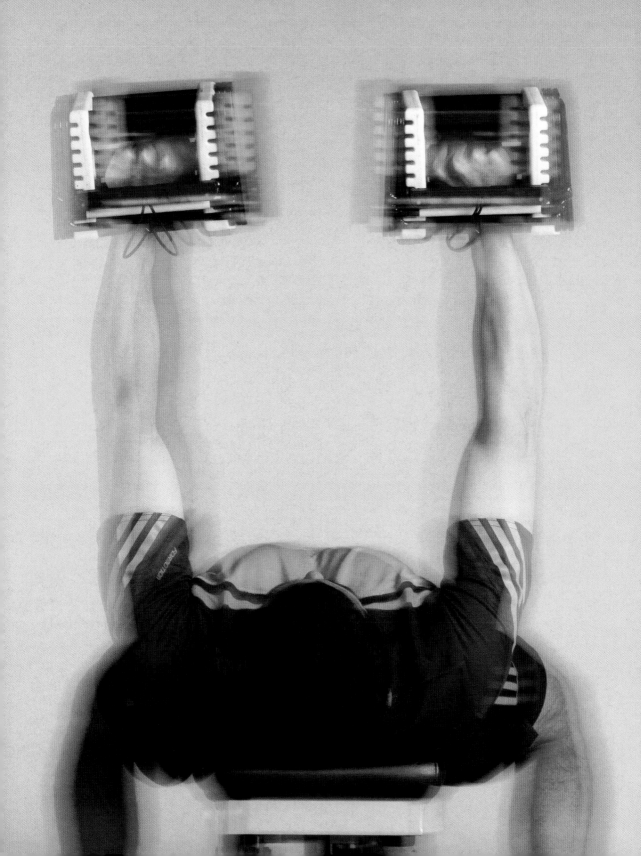

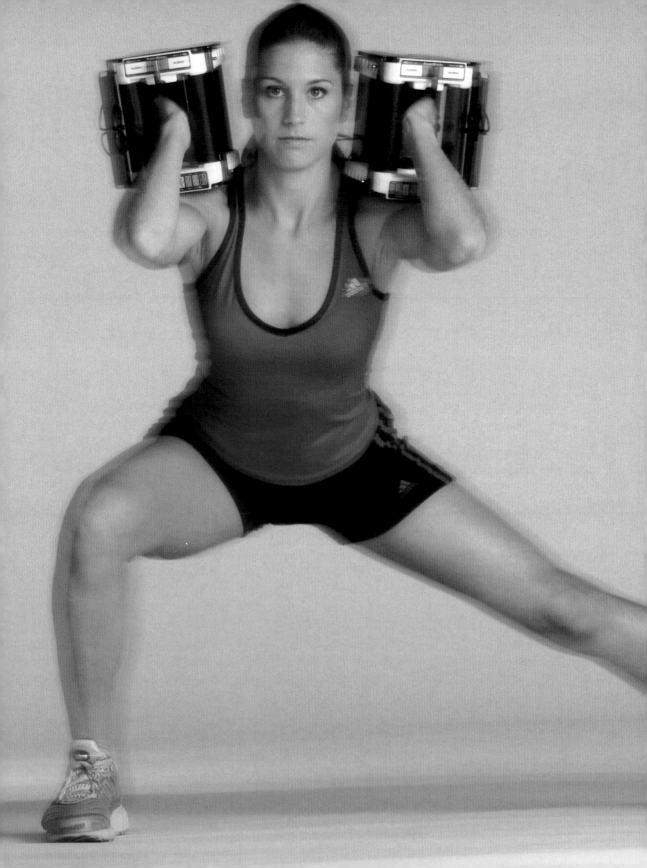

PART 4

THE CORE ENDURANCE WORKOUT

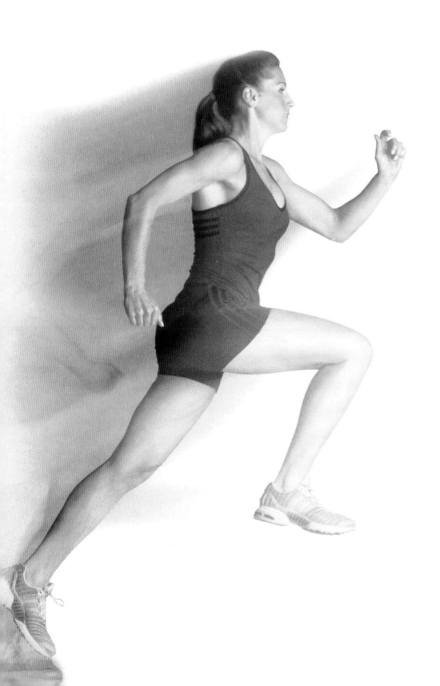

CHAPTER 9

THE
CORE ENDURANCE WORKOUT:
AN INTRODUCTION

W e've given you a lot of information in the first three sections. We know you can handle it, but if you're like me, you're probably wondering how you're going to fit it all into your hectic schedule. The goal with Core Performance Endurance (CPE) is to provide simple solutions that will allow everyone from novices to elite endurance athletes to maximize their return on the time invested.

How do we do that? We're going to organize this entire system into three themed training sessions: power, strength, and regeneration.

Within each of these sessions, you will find two levels (1 and 2). Within each of the two levels, you will find three stages (A, B,

and C). I don't break this down in terms of weeks or months. This is not a quick-fix, 12-week system. I want this to act as the foundation for the remainder of your active life, which hopefully will be the remainder of your life, period.

The levels will consist of similar movements and exercises, but the key is their *progressions*. In Level 1, for instance, we will take our core fundamental movement patterns and begin at the basic level. In Level 2, we will take the same exercises and make them slightly more challenging by progressing the movement, changing the proprioceptive demands, or adding a degree of complexity to give you greater return on investment for that particular exercise.

Just as we talked about everything in this program leading to greater efficiency, we want the workout to provide greater exercise economy as you progress from one level to the next. As you advance in the CPE system, some of the exercises you do in Level 2 might equate to two to three exercises you did in earlier levels. In that way, you get more benefit in less time.

This is the long-term performance solution to a time-crunched world. It's like anything else in life. There used to be a time where if we wanted to make a phone call, we had to locate and use a slow rotary phone and then consult a phone book or directory assistance. Now, the process can be as simple as flipping open your voice-activated cell phone.

Every other aspect of your life has advanced with technology, enabling you to accomplish more in less time. Why should training your body be any different?

You'll notice that each training day (power,

strength, regeneration) will consist of a few exercise units, namely the ones we discussed in the last section: (Movement Prep, Prehab, Elasticity, Strength, and Energy System Development, or ESD). I want you to complete these exercises, ideally in the specific order in which they're listed on your training plan.

You can do this at any point in the day. Ideally, you'll go through everything in one session, but with today's hectic lifestyles, you might find that it's easier to do the first two units in the morning and complete the third unit at lunchtime or after work. Either way, make sure that you over the course of the day go through the order that is prescribed.

If you're pressed for time, simply cut the number of sets to one, if that's what it takes to fit all the exercises in on that day. Consistency is what will lead to long-term success. Don't waste a lot of emotional energy worrying that you didn't get all of the sets done in one day. We're going to be satisfied with taking small, consistent steps toward our goal.

Ideally, it's best to get the whole workout all done at once. But no matter how you break it up or, if necessary, abbreviate it, invest this minimum amount of time. You owe it to your body. As an endurance athlete, you know what a tremendous return you receive by investing in yourself. Make this necessary investment, and the results will be tenfold. The Core Performance Endurance system will fit into or around your existing routines.

Again, don't get defeated. Some days will be more challenging than others. I travel frequently on business, and there are times when the end of the day comes, and it dawns on me that I haven't done anything. There's no hotel gym, my room is tiny, and it's nearly time for bed. But I still can step out into the hallway and do some Movement Prep, which, of course, I could easily have done in the morning.

The Core Performance system was designed to help you meet the demands of life. So we need to realize that sometimes we have to make allowances. It's okay.

If there's a large gap between when you perform the Movement Prep warmup routine and the other units, you might need to revisit a few Movement Prep exercises to get your body out of hibernation. Think of it as rebooting your computer.

Just as there are progressions in each of the two levels (1 and 2), there are progressions in each of the stages (A through C). At each stage, there's an increase in the amount of work you do, either an additional set or reps, that will make the workout more demanding. So the demand on your body increases as you progress from level to level and as you move from stage to stage.

You'll know when you're ready to advance a stage when you can perform the exercises for the prescribed number of repetitions perfectly in the allotted amount of time. When you master Stage C, completing the number of repetitions with perfect form in the allotted time, you're ready to jump to the next level.

When you advance to Level 2, you may not find the same number of sets and reps. That's by design. We're going to give your body and mind a chance to learn and master these more challenging progressions. From there, we'll progress through Stages A, B, and C, eventually making it to Level 3, which you can find at www.coreperformance.com/endurance.

When you arrive here, you'll have mastered some movements that many of your endurance-training friends will not have the ability to do. You'll marvel at how far you've come.

If family, work, or other life events knock you off the system, don't worry. That's part of the game of sports and life. What will make you a champion is getting right back up, dusting yourself off, and hopping back into the system.

Should that happen, it's best to start back at Level 1, Stage A, even if it's just for one workout apiece of 1-A, 1-B, and 1-C. Progress through Level 2 at the same pace until you feel challenged. This will allow you to pick up safely where you left off. Too often, people make the mistake of getting knocked off the horse and jumping right back on where they left off. That only leads to frustration, if not injury.

Before we discuss the details of the power, strength, and regeneration sessions, let's take a moment to do some planning. The foundation of this system is how well you plan. CPE will allow you to complete the proper training sessions, but the system has to be customized to your lifestyle. We all have different demands, goals, and abilities. If we plan properly, we can create a sound system to progress toward those goals.

Planning consists of manipulating the order of our three sessions, and we've kept it simple by giving you just three options. We've created planning tables with recommendations for basic and advanced programs, as well as for what to do during a race week. We always try to work from quality to quantity, meaning that we start with mastery of modest movements and workouts and then progress.

For the basic program, we want to incorporate more regeneration sessions at first. You'll notice a pattern of going from a power session to regeneration to strength and back to regeneration. That gives you a 1-to-1 ratio of work (power or strength) to rest (regeneration). As you improve, you can increase your work-to-regeneration ratios to 2-to-1 in favor of work. This is as far as I want you to take it, whether you're an amateur or an elite athlete.

Now, a few of you elite athletes will say that you're capable of much more than that. You're only fooling yourself. If you can endure more than 2 high-quality days back to back, you haven't experienced true high-quality or high-intensity training.

I've heard these same doubts from prominent world-class athletes at my Athletes' Performance Institutes. They quickly realize that this 2-to-1 work-to-regeneration ratio not only is ideal for maximum performance and recovery but also makes the most of their time.

Perhaps you have been willing your way through a long week. If you focus that same will and effort and execute the levels of quality and intensity on power days followed by a strength day at the highest intensity you're capable of, there's no way you could repeat a similar training session again on day 3. Even if you could, you wouldn't be able to do it more than twice.

Nor should you—it will only lead you to take constant withdrawals from your body's savings accounts, and that will leave you bankrupt through mental burnout, physical illness, or injury. Take my advice and focus your passionate intensity on each step and rep of these training sessions. Spend that effort so that when you're done with your sport or your power or strength session, you'll know that you executed it at a world-class level and that you had nothing more to give during any second of that session. At that point, you deserve to regenerate, to give your body time to recover the high-stress training days. Remember: Work + rest = success.

Your workdays are the stimulus for change. Regeneration days enable your body to improve. They facilitate recovery and give your body a chance to supercompensate and adapt to the stimulus it has received over the past few days.

A careful balance of work and regeneration will ensure that you don't under-recover and end up overtrained. It will keep you from improperly investing your hard effort.

Now let's take a look at our three training sessions in detail.

POWER DAYS

Today's theme is *power*. Power sessions consist of three exercise units, along with some ESD guidelines to help you organize specific techniques and tactics for your endurance sport. Our goal is not to be your endurance coach but to give you more tools to complement your endurance training programs.

The first unit in the power sessions is Movement Prep. You'll have 7 minutes to complete this unit. Movement Prep will increase your body's core temperature, elongate muscles actively and symmetrically, improve your balance and proprioception, and prepare you for the upcoming movement demands.

Movement Prep also helps you take a quick inventory as you boot up your body's computer system to see whether anything is out of the ordinary, such as a tight or painful muscle or joint. You'll have 7 minutes to perform one set of each of the five exercises. They will focus on your balance, stability, and mobility.

The Movement Prep exercises will also include some dynamic marching and skipping exercises. These allow you to feel elasticity developing through your body, and they prepare you for more intense elasticity movements to come.

Next, we'll have a Prehab unit, which contains five exercises to target the hips, torso, and shoulders. You'll strengthen and stabilize these pillar parts, activating them and protecting them from injury. By doing this, you'll put your body in the most advantageous position to perform the upcoming movement skills safely and efficiently. You'll have 10 minutes to perform two sets of each of the five exercise progressions in Prehab.

The third power unit is Elasticity. You'll have 12 minutes to do two sets of three exercises. These initially will focus on your ability to decelerate and stabilize some very simple movements. We'll then progress in these movements to become more dynamic until the end of Level 2, where you will train your body to be reactive, much like a springy Superball that stores and releases tremendous energy as it bounces. Soon you'll start to feel this sensation in every stride or stroke of your endurance training.

We've also included some ESD guidelines, all geared toward power. Focus on activities that require greater speed, elasticity, cardiovascular power, and leg power. You'll have between 4 and 10 repetitions of various intervals ranging from 30 seconds to 1 minute of intense work followed by intervals of 1-to-3, 1-to-2, or 1-to-1 work-to-rest ratios. Take your current training program and apply these guidelines so you perform complementary endurance training that fits your power goals for the day.

The complete power workout, excluding your endurance training, should take no more than 30 minutes. If you're pressed for time, you can complete the routine in less than 20 minutes by doing just one set of Prehab exercises, which will activate your muscles, and one set of Elasticity, to activate your central nervous system. That way, you'll still be able to get the most out of your upcoming endurance activity.

STRENGTH DAYS

Strength sessions will consist of just two units, each having two levels and three stages. The first is Movement Prep. You'll have 7 minutes to complete one set of five Movement Prep exercises.

Compared with the power session, these Movement Prep exercises focus more on mobility, stability, and strength. There are various lunges—forward, lateral, and drop—that will open the hip capsules, stretching and stabilizing the surrounding musculature from the hips all the way to the lower back. We'll pair this with a progression of "hand-walks" that will open up the calves and hamstrings, provide shoulder and rotary torso stability, and increase stride length.

The next unit in our strength day will be Energy System Development, or ESD. Go directly from Movement Prep to your endurance workout. The ESD guidelines will help develop your cardio strength. You'll either work at race pace or at a pace to develop base strength and your lactate threshold. So, look for a hill around your neighborhood with a grade between 3 and 10 percent that will take you between 4 and 8 minutes to navigate.

You'll have two levels and three stages, with heart rate zones between 55 and 85 percent. Intervals will range from 3 to 5 minutes of moderate intensity and build up to 5 minutes of hard intensity, ranging from a 1-to-2 work-to-rest ratio down to a 1-to-1 ratio. This will require you to put your hard hat on and go to work, but it will also allow you to develop that lactate threshold as an added weapon in your endurance training arsenal.

The actual strength circuit should take no more than 20 minutes. You will have seven exercises to perform in a circuit, meaning you'll go from one set of the first exercise to the next, all the way through all seven exercises. You'll then start back over with the first exercise, for a second time through the circuit.

The strength workout requires minimal equipment. Everything you need will fit in an exercise bag or bike box. You should be able to do this routine at home or wherever your profession or sport takes you around the world. You'll need access either to a cable or to a system such as the GoFit Pro Gym-in-a-Bag, which attaches to the back of any door. It's light, compact, and easy to travel with and store.

We'll also use the Valslide, a valuable slideboard device that improves stability, mobility, and strength. As with everything in the Core Performance system, if you don't have the means to acquire the optimal equipment, you can find simple substitutions around the house. Instead of a Valslide, you can use any slick surface such as hardwood, linoleum, or tile floors. You could even use carpeting if you put one foot over a clipboard or manila folder—place your foot on the object and slide over the carpet—though the Valslide is compact and perfect to take on the go.

These slideboard exercises not only will make you stronger, they'll also release tight muscles. The slideboard leg curl is one of the best all-around exercises for your glutes, hamstrings, calves, and lower back. It also provides an active stretch of the hip flexors and quads. The split and lunge positions that you'll assume are especially useful for stretching out all the muscles in your hips.

As you progress, you'll notice that these movements feel more related to movements you perform in your sport, which is exactly the point. This program is geared toward helping you re-establish and build upon the core fundamental movement patterns you were born with but have lost over time because of too much training, excessive screen time, or simply the demands of life.

Two of the primary exercises will be what we call "chopping" and its opposite movement, "lifting." These will require you to have stability from your feet all the way through your head. From this stable base, your muscles can generate force, whether you're in a vertical position (running), a horizontal position (swimming), or a combination of both (riding). You should feel tall through your torso, locking in stability and then moving your limbs around this stable foundation. The less movement here, the better.

You'll notice that some of these movements will attack small stabilizer muscles you didn't know you had. You'll feel small muscles burning in the bottoms of your feet, shoulders, and hips. We'll condition these muscles so that you won't even be aware of what a great job they're doing to help you generate force.

You'll have additional exercises for hip stability that will employ a cable or exercise bands. These will improve foot strength as well as hip stability. You will focus on the proper movement patterns with the moving leg attached to the cable. Soon, you'll realize that the load-bearing leg on the ground is burning from the arch you are trying to make in your foot in order to balance all the way up to your hip cuff.

You'll also be doing some leg curl exercises using the Valslide, which will act as a great activation and strengthening routine for the glutes, hamstrings, and calves. The leg curls will also bring about long-term flexibility gains in your hip flexors and quads. The leg curl movement pulls you into an active hip flexor and quad stretch by firing your glutes and hamstrings. It actually reprograms your mind to create balance in this region for long-term flexibility gains.

No strength workout would be complete without some form of squatting and upper-body pushing that requires great pillar strength and shoulder stability.

With the strength session, you can do Movement Prep followed by your endurance workout for the day, perhaps early, and then complete your strength circuit, either immediately after your ESD or (preferably) sometime later that day, after your body has recovered. Or, if you are doing the split session, another option is to do Movement Prep and Strength in the morning and ESD in the evening, since your body will be recovered.

If you feel that you already have great endurance and have been doing this for some time, you'll receive far greater improvement by going from Movement Prep immediately to your Strength circuit. Your stabilizing and propulsive strength might have more potential for improvement. Our goal with the CPE system is to identify and then attack your limiting factors.

By doing Movement Prep and then the Strength circuit, you'll receive a great return. There's far more upside to be found in this strength and stability training than, say, if you just took the same amount of time and added more running, riding, or swimming.

If strength is your limiting factor, do your Strength circuit before endurance training so you'll have more energy to put into the Strength routine. You'll get results more rapidly, which will result in a greater impact on your endurance performance. Your legs may feel a little heavy initially, but remember that the goal with endurance training is to hold the proper movement patterns and biomechanics at a pace and at a heart rate at which you can maintain those mechanics. Gradually, you can build up legs with quality endurance work.

Remember the long-term goal. Can you execute proper biomechanics to achieve high-quality movement, and then achieve high-quality endurance? Develop the energy system that corresponds to the Strength unit, which is lactate threshold training, and your heart rate and lactate threshold will be significantly challenged. You might feel tired and might run slower times than when you were fresh, but that's okay; we're achieving the desired results from proper mechanics and attacking the appropriate heart rate zone.

Your complete strength workout, not including your ESD, should take a maximum of 27 minutes. If you're time-crunched, you should be able to complete the routine in 15 to 17 minutes by doing just one set of each Strength circuit exercise.

One final note on strength training equipment: We would love to be able to share with you the power and benefit of using a medicine ball in your workout. "Med" balls are a tremendous aid in taking your performance to the next level. Unfortunately, most gyms do not offer the concrete block wall that's needed to perform these workouts properly. If you'd like to learn more about med ball training, which is especially useful for swimming, running, and riding, please visit www.coreperformance.com/endurance, go to the "Core Store," and locate our programs for running, riding, swimming, and triathlon.

REGENERATION DAYS

Today's theme is *regeneration*. This should carry through the entire day, from the final rep of the previous day's training session. It includes your mindset at work and your personal time. That's your window of opportunity—from the moment you finish your workout until your next power or strength session or competition.

We're creating a lifestyle, and "regen" is not only a workout but also a mindset. It allows us to recharge our batteries mentally and physically so that we're poised to create more energy and sustain that energy in all aspects of life. If you don't make regeneration a priority, your body will go into a downward spiral. Ultimately, it will shut down through injury or illness until you make the time to recover. Regeneration is a more enjoyable and efficient way to achieve a superior result. The goal of regeneration, as with the rest of the CPE program, is to help you get more out of your routines in less time.

Regeneration sessions are structured differently from the power and strength sessions. We've created a menu for you to address the most common crucial areas for endurance athletes. There are categories for your lower legs, hips, torso, and shoulders. Pick one based on whichever area needs attention the most. We're going to facilitate recovery through "active-isolated stretching," or AIS, as well as through static stretching, and we'll complement this with targeted self-massage. We'll show you how to target key pressure points to remove knots and spasms.

You'll self-massage by using a foam roll, improve flexibility with active-isolated stretching, and address the key pressure points in your problem areas.

The quality of your tissue and the demands of your past few training days and weeks will dictate how long you need to spend on self-massage. It could last anywhere from 5 to 30 minutes.

You'll also do three to five Movement Prep exercises and a regeneration "flush," an ESD workout at about 60 to 65 percent of your lactate threshold (220 minus your age). The entire regeneration session will last between 20 and 60 minutes, depending on which level of the program you're in.

The lower-impact regeneration activities will allow your body to flush itself out, adding some necessary volume and, potentially, distance while minimizing stress to the central nervous system and tissue. Even if you're feeling terrific on regeneration days, it's important that you don't push it and add

intensity. With regeneration, we're going to recharge, so you'll be recovered and fired up for your next power or strength day.

Before undergoing your regeneration flush, be sure to do the three to five Movement Prep exercises that you feel you need. You might find that you need to break out your flush either before or after your tissue management (massage, foam roll, etc.), and that's okay. You may find it easiest to get the tissue portion of the regeneration day done first thing in the morning and do your flush later that afternoon—or vice versa. Sometimes, it's most convenient to get the flush done in the morning and the tissue maintenance in the evening as you relax in front of television. You can also do tissue maintenance daily, after your training session.

CHAPTER 9 SUMMARY: The Core Endurance Workout is organized into power, strength, and regeneration days. Power days consist of three exercise units, along with some Energy System Development (ESD) guidelines, to give you more tools to complement your endurance training program. Strength days consist of Movement Prep, which focuses on developing mobility and stability, and ESD, which builds cardio strength. Finally, regeneration helps you actively recover from the other more strenuous days and enables you to come back stronger.

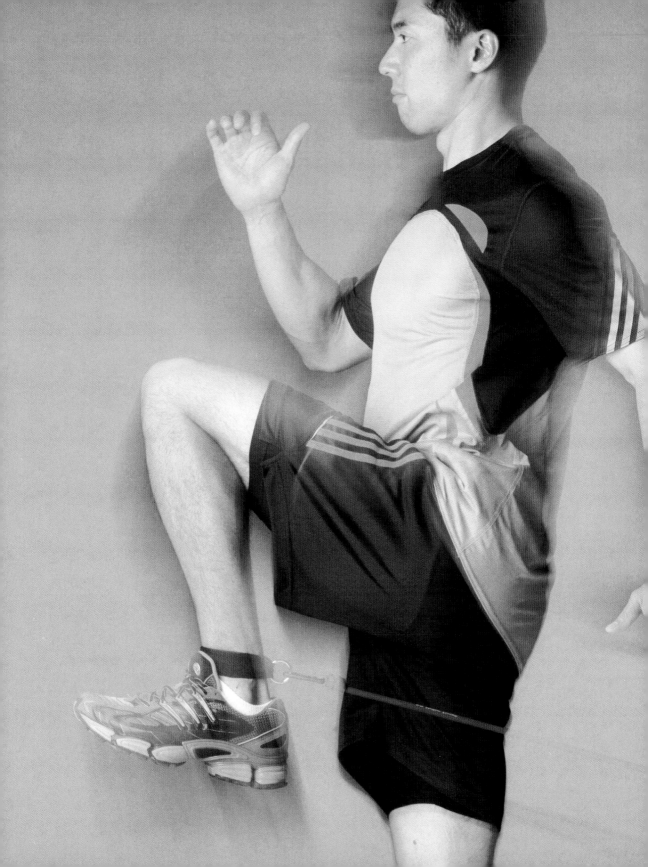

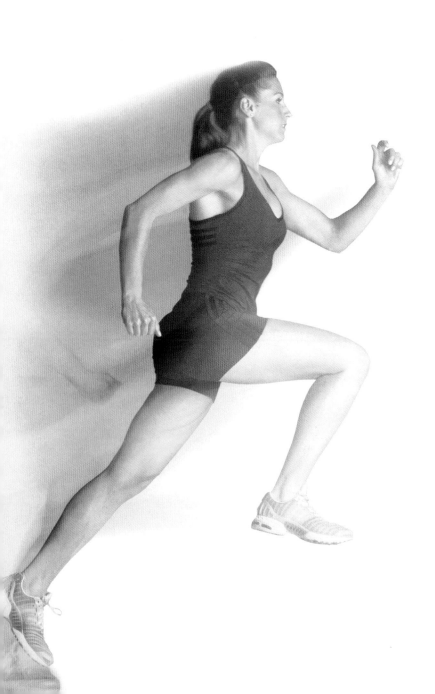

CHAPTER 10

CORE MOVEMENTS

Before we organize our workouts into power, strength, and regeneration days, let's take a unit-by-unit look at each exercise.

If some of these exercises seem awkward or difficult at first, don't worry. You'll adapt quickly. One of the exciting parts of the Core Performance Endurance program is experiencing these "a-ha" moments as you discover these new methods of improving performance for yourself.

REVERSE 90/90 STRETCH

STARTING POSITION:

Holding a pad with both hands, lie faceup on the ground, your right knee bent to 90 degrees and your left leg crossed over the right.

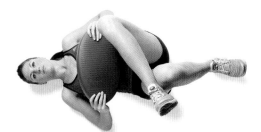

PROCEDURE:

Roll over on your right side, pinning the pad between your left knee and the ground, and hold your left arm straight in the air. Keeping your left arm in the air, lift your right arm as high as possible. Hold for 2 seconds and return to the starting position. Repeat for the prescribed number of reps and switch sides.

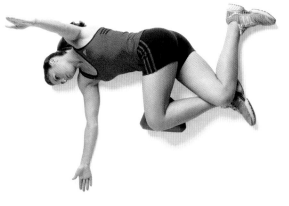

COACHING KEY:

Keep pressure against the pad with the knee of your top leg. Lift your arm only as far as you can while keeping your knee down. Exhale as you stretch.

YOU SHOULD FEEL:

A stretch in your torso and tension in your groin.

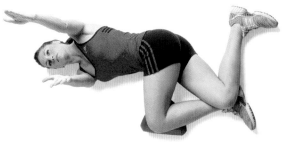

INVERTED HAMSTRING STRETCH (IN PLACE)

STARTING POSITION:

Stand on one leg with perfect posture, your arms raised to 90 degrees and your thumbs up, and your shoulder blades back and down.

PROCEDURE:

Keeping a straight line between your ear and ankle, bend over at the waist and elevate your other leg behind you. When you feel a stretch, return to the standing position by contracting your glutes and hamstring. Repeat on the same leg for the prescribed number of reps, then switch legs.

COACHING KEY:

Keep your back flat and your hips parallel to the ground. Maintain a straight line from your ear through your hip, knee, and ankle. Try not to let your foot touch the ground between repetitions.

YOU SHOULD FEEL:

A stretch in your hamstrings.

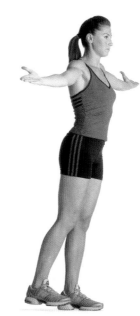

FORWARD LUNGE, ELBOW TO INSTEP (CRAWLING)

STARTING POSITION:

Stand with your back straight and your arms at your sides.

PROCEDURE:

Step forward into a lunge with your left foot. Place your right hand on the ground and your left elbow to the inside of your left foot, and hold the stretch for 1 to 2 seconds. Place your left hand outside of your foot and push your hips toward the sky. Drop your hips and crawl into the next repetition with the other leg. Continue for the prescribed number of reps.

COACHING KEY:

Keep your back knee off the ground. Contract your back glute during the stretch.

YOU SHOULD FEEL:

A stretch in your groin, your back leg hip flexor, and your front leg glute and hamstring.

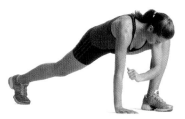

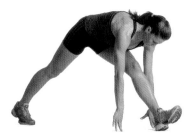

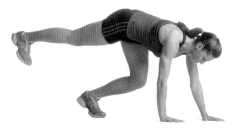

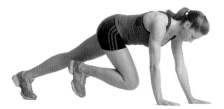

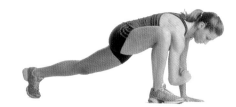

KNEE HUG (IN PLACE)

STARTING POSITION:

Stand with your back straight and your arms at your sides.

PROCEDURE:

Lift your right knee to your chest and grab below the knee with your hands. Pull your right knee as close to your chest as you can while contracting your left glute. Return to the starting position and repeat on the other side. Continue, alternating sides, for the prescribed number of reps.

COACHING KEY:

Keep your chest up. Contract the glute of the leg you are standing on.

YOU SHOULD FEEL:

A stretch in the glute and hamstring of your front leg and in the hip flexor of your back leg.

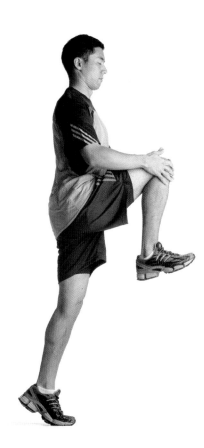

PILLAR MARCH (MOVING)

STARTING POSITION:

Stand with your back straight and your arms at your sides.

PROCEDURE:

Lift the knee and foot of one leg, as you lift the opposite arm. Drive your foot down to the ground as you lift your opposite foot and knee and the other arm. Alternate and repeat, moving forward.

COACHING KEY:

Maintain perfect posture. Keep your toes pulled up to your shins. Push the trailing foot down and back through the ground and let your hip go into full extension. Initiate the movement from your glutes. Drive your elbow back as the opposite leg attacks the ground.

YOU SHOULD FEEL:

Movement everywhere—this is a total-body exercise.

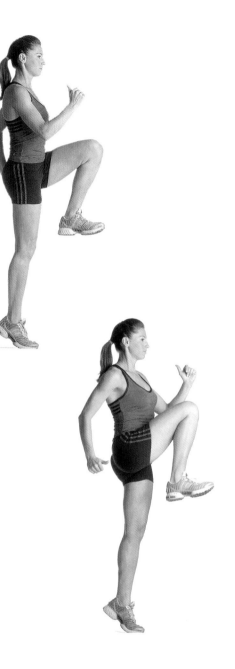

BACKWARD LUNGE WITH LATERAL FLEXION (IN PLACE)

STARTING POSITION:

Stand with your back straight and your arms at your sides.

PROCEDURE:

Step backward with your right foot into the lunge, your left foot forward, then contract your right glute. Reach your right hand overhead and laterally crunch your torso to the left, reaching your left hand to the ground. Return to the starting position and repeat on the opposite side. Alternate for the desired number of reps.

COACHING KEY:

Maintain your posture throughout the movement. Contract your back glute during the stretch. Keep your front knee behind your toes. Don't let your back knee touch the ground. Keep your chest up and fire your front glute as you return to the starting position.

YOU SHOULD FEEL:

Stretching in the hip flexor of your back leg, in the glute and groin area of your front leg, and in the lateral muscles of your torso.

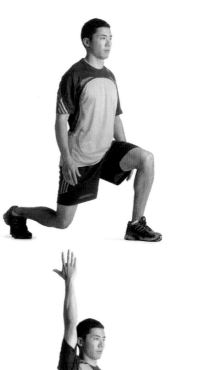

LEG CRADLE

STARTING POSITION:

Stand with your back straight, your knees unlocked, and your arms at your sides.

PROCEDURE:

Lift your right foot off the ground and squat back and down while standing on your left leg. Lift your right knee to your chest, placing your right hand under the knee and your left hand under the ankle. Pull your right leg as close as you can to your chest into a gentle stretch while contracting your left glute. Now step forward with your right foot. Alternate feet and repeat for the prescribed number of reps.

COACHING KEY:

Keep your chest up. Contract the glute of the leg you are standing on.

YOU SHOULD FEEL:

Stretching on the outside of your hip in your front leg and in the hip flexor of your back leg.

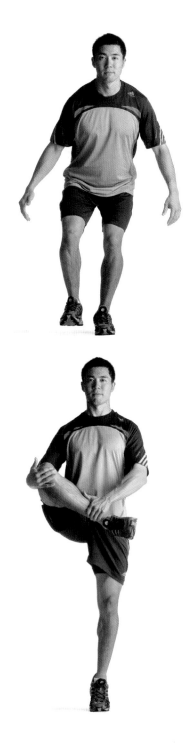

QUADRUPED POSTERIOR ROCKING

STARTING POSITION:

Get down on all fours with your hands under your shoulders and your knees under your hips.

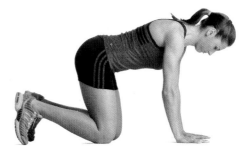

PROCEDURE:

Pull your belly button in toward your spine while maintaining a natural curve in your lower back. Move your hips backward until you start feeling your pelvis rotating. Return to the starting position and repeat for the prescribed number of reps.

COACHING KEY:

Draw your belly button in without losing the curve in your lower back or feeling your rib cage expanding. You should be able to breathe normally. Try to hold your pelvis still throughout the range of motion.

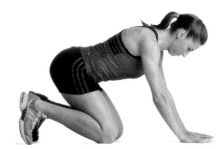

YOU SHOULD FEEL:

Compression in the front of your hips. This works your lower back and mobilizes your hips.

INVERTED HAMSTRING STRETCH (BACKWARD)

STARTING POSITION:

Stand on one leg with perfect posture, arms raised to 90 degrees and shoulder blades back and down.

PROCEDURE:

Keeping a straight line between the ear and ankle, bend over at the waist and elevate your opposite leg behind you. When you feel a stretch, return to the standing position by contracting your glute and hamstring, stepping back into the next step with your opposite leg. Repeat the motion, alternating legs with each step backward for the prescribed number of reps.

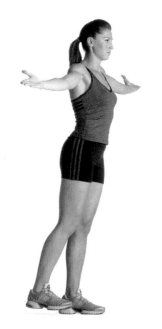

COACHING KEY:

Keep the knee of the leg you are standing on slightly bent. Keep your back flat and your hips parallel to the ground. Maintain a straight line from your ear through your hip, knee, and ankle of your leg in the air. Try not to let your raised foot touch the ground between repetitions.

YOU SHOULD FEEL IT:

Stretching your hamstrings and challenging your balance.

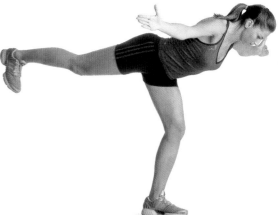

FORWARD LUNGE, ELBOW TO INSTEP (WALKING)

STARTING POSITION:

Stand with your back straight and your arms at your sides.

PROCEDURE:

Step forward into a lunge with your left foot. Place your right hand on the ground and your left elbow to the inside of your left foot, and hold the stretch for 1 to 2 seconds. Place your left hand outside of your foot and push your hips toward the sky. Drop your hips and lift your chest and step into the next repetition with the other leg. Continue for the prescribed number of reps.

COACHING KEY:

Keep your back knee off the ground. Contract your back glute during the stretch. Lead with your chest as you step into the next repetition.

YOU SHOULD FEEL:

A stretch in your groin, your back leg hip flexor, and your front leg glute and hamstring.

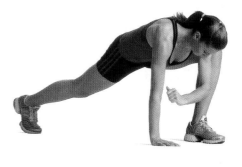

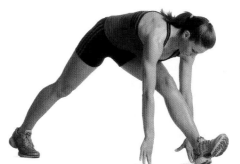

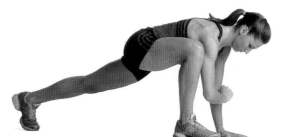

KNEE HUG (MOVING)

STARTING POSITION:

Stand with your back straight and your arms at your sides.

PROCEDURE:

Lift your right foot off the ground and squat back and down while standing on your left leg. Lift your right knee to your chest and grab below the knee with your hands. Pull your right knee as close as you can to your chest while contracting your left glute. Step forward and repeat on the other side. Continue alternating sides and moving forward for the prescribed number of reps.

COACHING KEY:

Keep your chest up. Contract the glute of the leg you are standing on. Do not let your knee slide forward during the squat.

YOU SHOULD FEEL IT:

Stretching the glute and hamstring of your front leg and the hip flexor of your back leg.

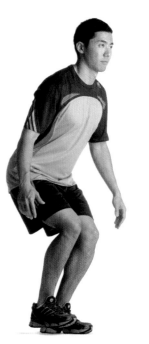

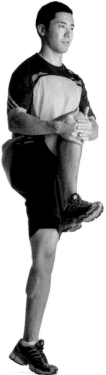

PILLAR SKIP (IN PLACE)

STARTING POSITION:

Stand with your back straight and your arms at your sides.

PROCEDURE:

Lift the knee and foot of one leg as you lift your opposite arm. Drive your foot down to the ground, generating a double foot contact as your opposite foot and knee begin to lift. Alternate legs and arms, repeating for the prescribed number of reps while remaining in place.

COACHING KEY:

Maintain perfect posture. Keep your toes pulled up to your shins. Push your foot through to the ground with your hips going into full extension. Initiate the movement from your glutes. Drive your elbow back as the opposite leg attacks the ground.

YOU SHOULD FEEL IT:

Working your entire body.

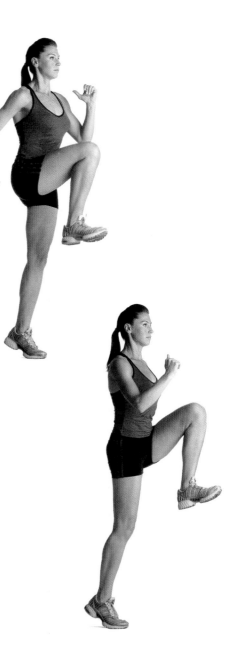

BACKWARD LUNGE WITH LATERAL FLEXION (MOVING)

STARTING POSITION:

Stand with your back straight and your arms at your sides.

PROCEDURE:

Step forward with your left foot, then contract your right glute. Reach your right hand overhead and laterally crunch your torso to the left, reaching your left hand to the ground. Hold perfect posture as you step backward into the next lunge. Repeat the movement on the opposite side, alternating sides for the desired number of reps.

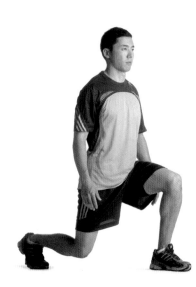

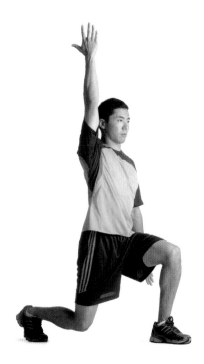

COACHING KEY:

Maintain your posture throughout the movement. Contract your back glute during the stretch. Keep your front knee behind your toes. Don't let your back knee touch the ground. Keep your chest up as you step backward into the next rep.

YOU SHOULD FEEL:

Stretching in the hip flexor of your back leg, in the glute and groin area of your front leg, and in the lateral muscles of your torso.

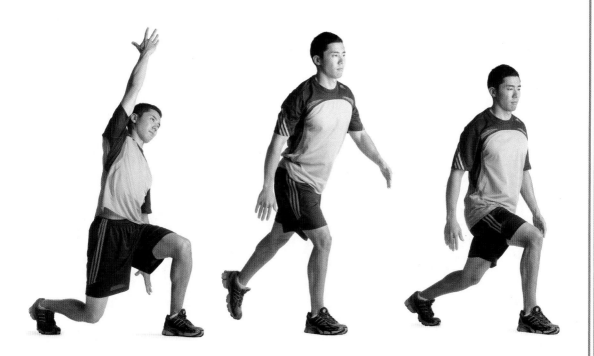

DROP LUNGE

STARTING POSITION:

Stand with your back straight and your hands clasped at chest height.

PROCEDURE:

Reach your left foot behind and 2 feet beyond the outside of your right foot. Square your hips back to the starting position and sit back and down into a squat. Now stand and step laterally with your right foot, repeating the stretch on same side. Continue for the prescribed number of reps and then reverse directions.

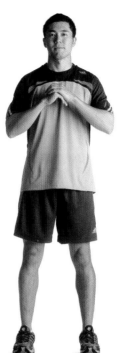

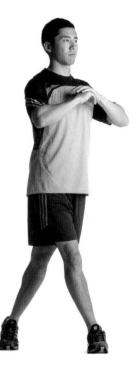

COACHING KEY:

Keep your chest up. Maintain weight on the heel of your front leg. Do not let your front knee slide over your toe.

YOU SHOULD FEEL:

Stretching in the outside of both hips.

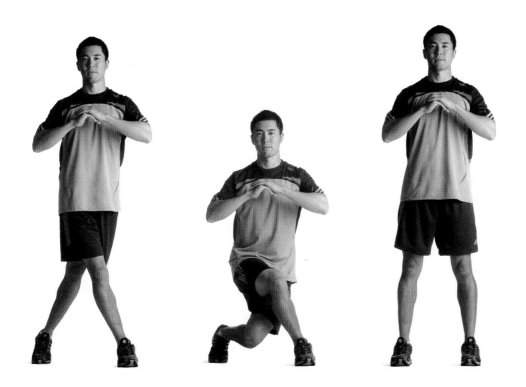

PILLAR BRIDGE FRONT

STARTING POSITION:

Lie facedown with your forearms on the ground under your chest.

PROCEDURE:

Push up off your elbows, supporting your weight on the forearms. Tuck your chin so that your head is in line with your body, and pull your toes toward your shins. Hold the position for the prescribed time.

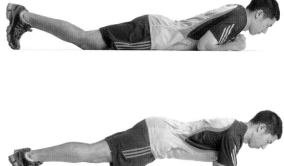

COACHING KEY:

Push your chest as far away from the ground as possible. Keep your belly button drawn in. Keep your head in line with your spine. Don't sag or bend. Do not round off your upper back.

YOU SHOULD FEEL IT:

Working your shoulders and core.

PILLAR BRIDGE LATERAL—FEET SPLIT

STARTING POSITION:

Lie on your side with your body in a straight line and your elbow under your shoulder, your feet split with the top leg forward.

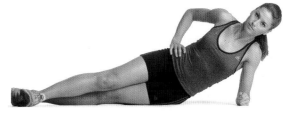

PROCEDURE:

Push your hip off the ground, creating a straight line from ankle to shoulder. Hold for the prescribed time. Switch sides and repeat.

COACHING KEY:

Push your torso away from the ground, keeping your tummy tight. Keep your head in line with your spine. Keep your hips pushed forward and your body straight. Maintain straight lines—no sagging or bending.

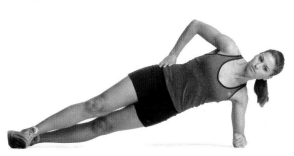

YOU SHOULD FEEL IT:

Working your shoulders and core.

GLUTE BRIDGE MARCHING (KNEE EXTENSION)

STARTING POSITION:

Lie faceup on the ground with your arms to your sides, your knees bent, and your heels on the ground.

PROCEDURE:

Lift your hips off the ground until your knees, hips, and shoulders are in a straight line. Hold the position while extending your left knee. Return your foot to the ground and repeat with your right knee. Repeat for the prescribed number of reps.

COACHING KEY:

Don't let your back hyperextend. Don't let your hips drop as your knee comes to your chest.

YOU SHOULD FEEL IT:

Working your glutes mostly and to a lesser degree your hamstrings and lower back.

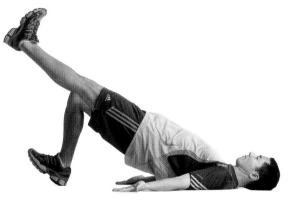

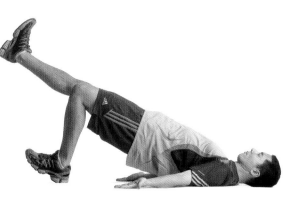

MINI BAND INTERNAL/EXTERNAL ROTATION

STARTING POSITION:

Stand with your feet slightly wider apart than your shoulders, your hips back and down, your back flat, and a mini band around your legs just above your knees.

PROCEDURE:

Keeping your left leg stationary, move your right knee in and out for the prescribed number of reps. Switch legs and repeat for the prescribed number of reps.

COACHING KEY:

Keep both feet flat on the ground. Keep your pelvis stable. Don't let the knee of your stationary leg drop in.

YOU SHOULD FEEL IT:

Working your glutes.

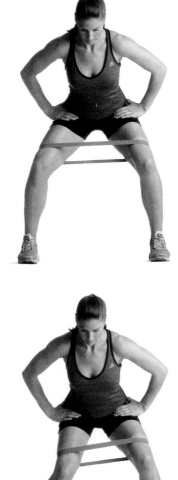

FOUR-WAY HIP CABLE

STARTING POSITION:

Stand facing a low pulley cable machine, your belly tight, an ankle strap attached to your right ankle.

PROCEDURE:

Extension: While maintaining good posture, slowly move your right leg backward, then slowly return to the starting position. Repeat for the prescribed number of reps.

Abduction: Turn 90 degrees clockwise and slowly move your right leg out from your body to the side, then back to your body, for the prescribed number of reps.

Flexion: Turn 90 degrees clockwise and slowly lift your knee in front of your body, then back down, for the prescribed number of reps.

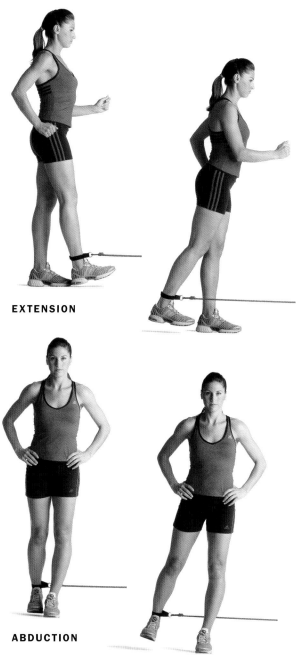

EXTENSION

ABDUCTION

Adduction: Turn 90 degrees clockwise and slowly move your straight leg toward and across your body, then back, for the prescribed number of reps. Switch legs and repeat all 4 movements.

COACHING KEY:

Try to remain balanced on one leg throughout the movements. Do not allow any motion to occur in your spine throughout the movements.

YOU SHOULD FEEL IT:

Working both hips and challenging your balance.

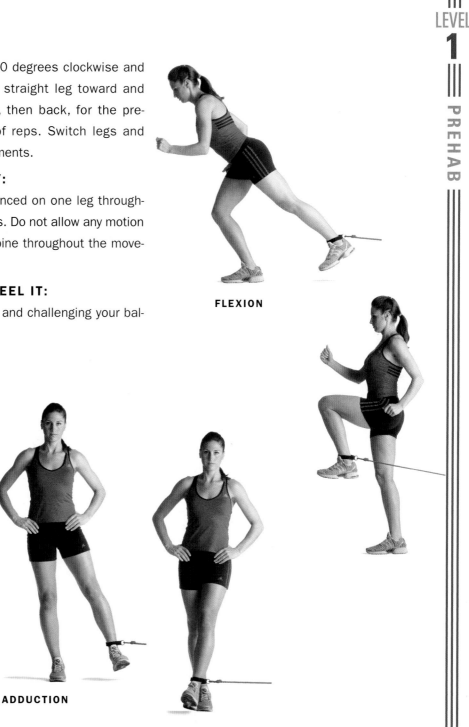

FLEXION

ADDUCTION

FLOOR *Y*s

STARTING POSITION:

Lie facedown on the floor with your bent arms raised slightly above shoulder height, to create a *Y*, with your torso and thumbs up (see inset).

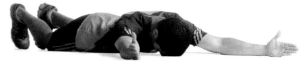

PROCEDURE:

Glide your shoulder blades toward your spine and lift your arms off the ground. Return to the starting position and repeat for the prescribed number of reps.

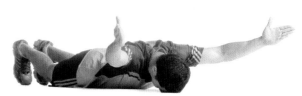

COACHING KEY:

Keep your stomach tight and your thumbs up. Move from the scapulae (shoulder blades), extending your shoulders and hands.

YOU SHOULD FEEL IT:

Working your shoulders and upper back.

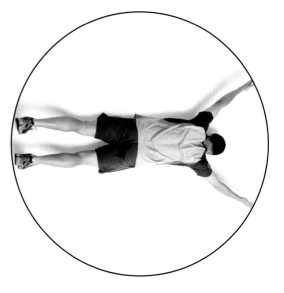

FRONT PILLAR WITH DIAGONAL ARM LIFT

STARTING POSITION:

Assume a pushup position with your feet wider than shoulder width apart.

PROCEDURE:

Without moving your torso, lift your left arm up and slightly to the left and hold for 1 to 2 seconds. Return to the starting position and repeat with your right arm (see inset). Repeat for the prescribed number of reps.

COACHING KEY:

Try to keep your weight even on both feet as your arm lifts. Do not let your trunk move as your arm leaves the ground. Keep your stomach tight throughout the movement.

YOU SHOULD FEEL IT:

Working your shoulders and trunk.

LATERAL PILLAR (ABDUCTION)

STARTING POSITION:

Lie on your side with your body in a straight line and your elbow under your shoulder, feet stacked.

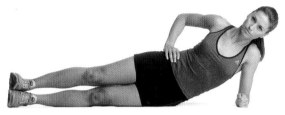

PROCEDURE:

Push your hip off the ground, creating a straight line from ankle to shoulder, keeping your head in line with your spine. Lift your top leg vertically while stabilizing the rest of your body, and lower back down in control. Repeat for the prescribed number of reps. Switch sides and repeat.

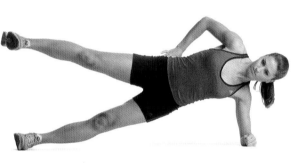

COACHING KEY:

Push your torso away from the ground, keeping your tummy tight. Keep your head in line with your spine. Keep your hips pushed forward and your body straight. Make sure both legs are straight, with toes up.

YOU SHOULD FEEL IT:

Working the shoulders, torso, and lateral hip stabilizers.

GLUTE BRIDGE MARCHING (HIP FLEXION)

STARTING POSITION:

Lie faceup on the ground with your arms to your sides, your knees bent, and your heels on the ground.

PROCEDURE:

Lift your hips off the ground until your knees, hips, and shoulders are in a straight line. Hold the position while lifting your left knee to your chest. Return your foot to the ground and repeat with your right knee. Continue for the prescribed number of reps.

COACHING KEY:

Do not let your back hyperextend. Do not let your hips drop as your knee comes to your chest.

YOU SHOULD FEEL IT:

Working mainly your glutes, and secondarily your hamstrings and lower back.

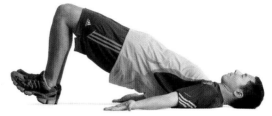

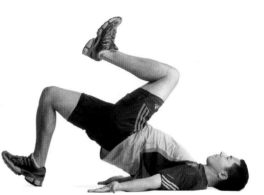

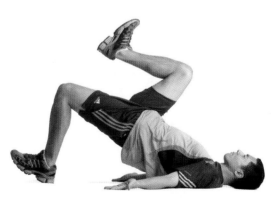

MINI BAND BENT-KNEE WALK

STARTING POSITION:

Stand in a quarter-squat position with your feet hip width apart and a mini band above your knees.

PROCEDURE:

Walk forward with small steps as your elbows drive back with each step. Continue for the prescribed number of reps on each foot.

COACHING KEY:

Keep your chest up and your back flat. Keep your knees pushed apart and over your toes at all times. Keep tension on the mini band at all times.

YOU SHOULD FEEL IT:

Working your glutes.

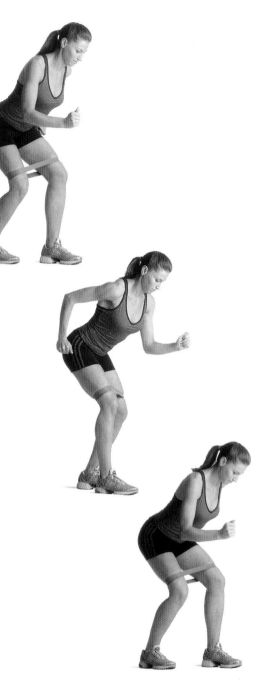

STANDING CABLE CROSSOVER

STARTING POSITION:

Stand with your hips perpendicular to a low cable pulley station with your left leg closest to the station, a cable attached to your left ankle.

PROCEDURE:

Balancing on your right leg, rotate your pelvis to the right while pulling your left foot up and across your body into a running crossover position. Slowly return to the starting position, maintaining your balance. Continue for the prescribed number of reps, then switch sides.

COACHING KEY:

Keep your toe pulled to your shin. Maintain good pillar position throughout the activity. Rotate around a central axis.

YOU SHOULD FEEL IT:

In the hip of your balancing leg and the hip flexors of your opposite leg.

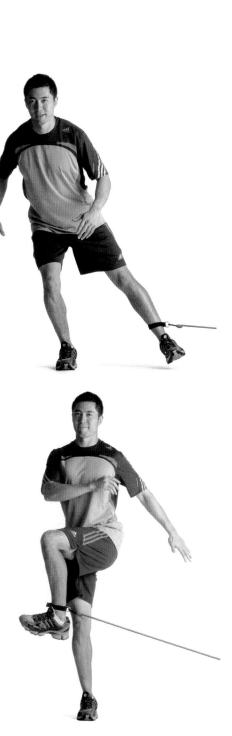

BENT-OVER *Ys* AND *Ls*

STARTING POSITION:

Stand bent over at the waist with your back flat and your chest up.

PROCEDURE:

Ys: Glide your shoulder blades back and down, then raise your arms over your head to form a Y. Return to the starting position and continue for the prescribed number of reps.

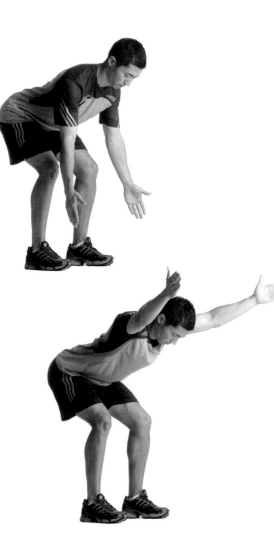

Ls: Glide your shoulder blades back and down, lift your elbows to the ceiling as they bend to 90 degrees, and rotate your hands toward the ceiling, palms down. Return to the starting position and continue for the prescribed number of reps.

COACHING KEY:

Initiate the movement with your shoulder blades, not your arms. On the *Y*, keep your thumbs up.

YOU SHOULD FEEL IT:

Working your shoulders and your upper and lower back.

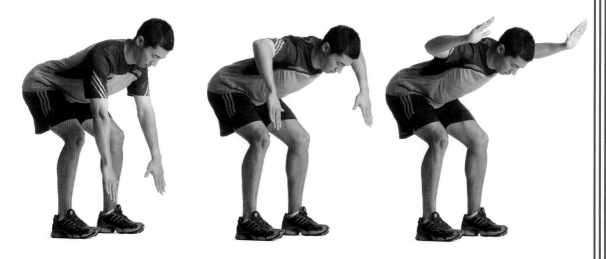

MINI BAND LATERAL BOUND—STABILIZATION

STARTING POSITION:

Stand on one leg with a mini band around both legs, above your knees.

PROCEDURE:

Load your hip and arms back and down. Now bound laterally, landing on the opposite foot, and hold for 3 seconds. Return to the starting position and repeat the bound to the other side. Continue for the prescribed number of reps.

COACHING KEY:

Use your hip and your arms to generate force. Bound for both distance and height and "stick" the landing. Land softly by absorbing the shock through your hip and keeping your feet straight ahead. Press laterally into the band with both legs to help maintain stability between bounds.

YOU SHOULD FEEL IT:

Working your hips and legs.

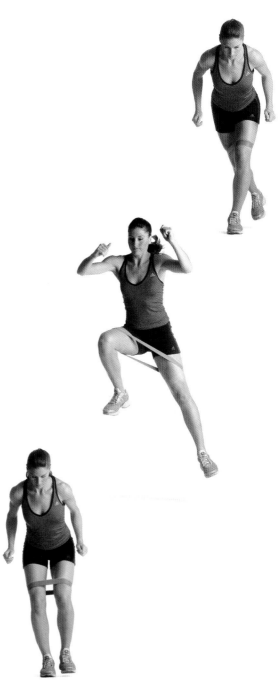

LINEAR BOX HOP

STARTING POSITION:

Stand on one leg facing a step box.

PROCEDURE:

Load your hip and arms back and down and hop forward onto the box. Hold a stable landing position for 3 seconds. Step off the box and continue the drill on the same leg for the prescribed reps, then repeat on the other leg.

COACHING KEY:

Use your hip and arms to generate force. Land softly by absorbing the shock through your hip. Do not allow your knee to collapse to the inside upon takeoff or landing.

YOU SHOULD FEEL IT:

Working your hip and leg.

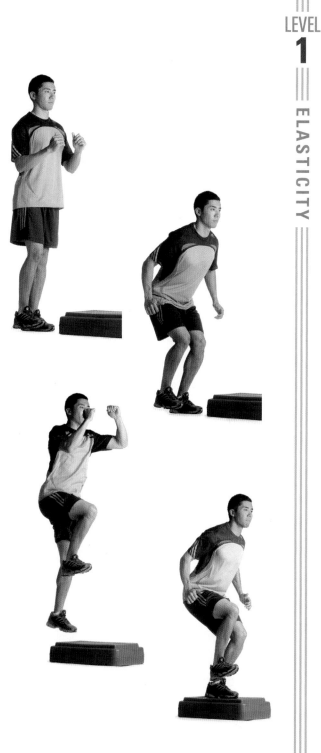

DROP SQUAT AND STABILIZE

STARTING POSITION:

Stand with your feet just outside of your shoulders, your elbows bent, and your arms up and fists level with your chin.

PROCEDURE:

Lift your feet off the ground and sit back and down into a squat position, keeping your knees behind your toes. As your hips drop into a squat position, raise your arms in front of you.

COACHING KEY:

Move with speed and stick the landing, keeping your chest up and back flat during the movement. Your feet should leave the ground during the movement. Do not allow your knees to collapse to the inside upon landing.

YOU SHOULD FEEL IT:

Working your hips and legs.

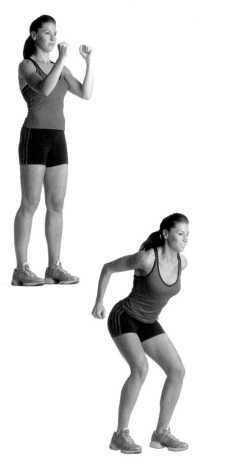

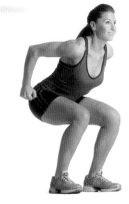

SQUAT JUMP—NON-COUNTERMOVEMENT

STARTING POSITION:

Stand with your feet just outside of your shoulders and your hands behind your head. Now sit back and down into a squat position, keeping your knees behind your toes.

PROCEDURE:

After holding the starting position for 3 seconds, jump vertically. Pull your toes to your shins in midair to prepare for landing. Land in the starting squat position, hold 3 seconds, and repeat.

COACHING KEY:

Keep your chest up during the jump and extend your hips completely. Land softly, with your hips back and down.

YOU SHOULD FEEL IT:

Working your hips, knees, and ankles.

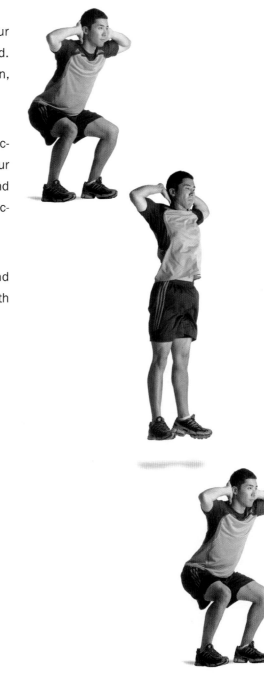

LATERAL BOUND—QUICK/STABILIZE

STARTING POSITION:

Stand on one leg and load your hip and arms back and down.

PROCEDURE:

Bound laterally, landing on the opposite foot. Without pausing, bound back to the other leg and hold 3 seconds. Continue for the prescribed number of reps, then switch sides.

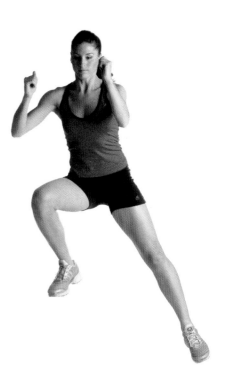
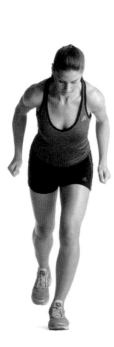

COACHING KEY:

Use your hip and arms to generate force. Bound for both distance and height. Anticipate the ground, minimizing contact time on the "quick" side. Land softly by absorbing the shock through your hip. Keep your stomach tight and your feet straight ahead throughout the movement.

YOU SHOULD FEEL IT:

Working your hips and legs.

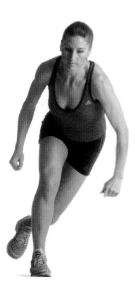
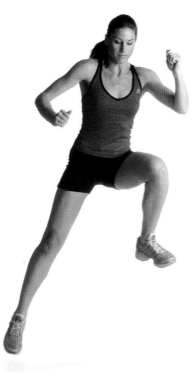
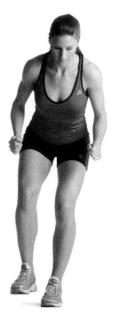

DOUBLE-CONTACT HURDLE HOP

STARTING POSITION:

Stand on one leg in front of a line of hurdles.

PROCEDURE:

Hop forward over one hurdle and land in a stable position. Quickly bounce on the landing foot, and on the second contact with the ground, hop over the next hurdle. Continue over the remaining hurdles. Repeat on the other leg.

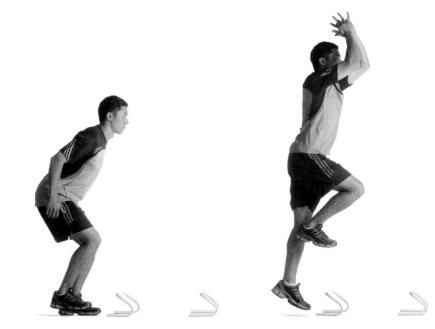

COACHING KEY:

Use your hip and arms to generate force. Land softly by absorbing the shock through your hip. Anticipate the ground on every contact, and try to minimize ground contact time following the second contact. Do not allow your knee to collapse to the inside upon takeoff or landing.

YOU SHOULD FEEL IT:

Working your hips and legs.

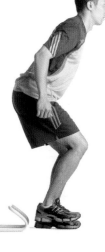

SQUAT JUMP—COUNTERMOVEMENT

STARTING POSITION:

Stand with your feet just outside of your shoulders and hands behind your head.

PROCEDURE:

Sit back and down into a squat position, keeping your knees behind your toes. Immediately jump vertically by extending through your hips. Pull your toes to your shins in midair to prepare for landing in the squat position. Reset to starting position and repeat.

COACHING KEY:

Do not pause at the bottom of the movement. Keep your chest up during the jump. Extend your hips completely during the jump.

YOU SHOULD FEEL IT:

Working your hips, knees, and ankles.

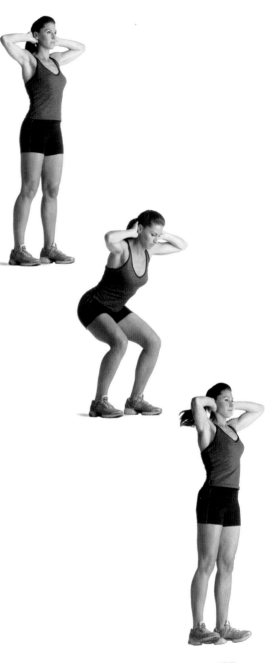

REACTIVE STEPUP

STARTING POSITION:

Stand with one foot flat on a box, your arms bent at the elbows to 90 degrees and cocked back.

PROCEDURE:

Jump vertically by throwing your arms up and exploding through your front leg, extending your hip, knee, and ankle. In the air, your front and back legs should exchange positions so that you land with the opposite foot on the box. Without pausing, immediately repeat the jump with the opposite leg. Continue for the prescribed number of reps.

COACHING KEY:

Throw your arms up but stop with your elbows at chin level. Land with your full foot on the box. Your torso should be leaning forward slightly upon landing, with your back leg slightly bent. Anticipate each landing to minimize contact time.

YOU SHOULD FEEL IT:

In your hips and legs.

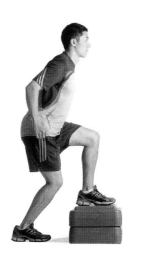
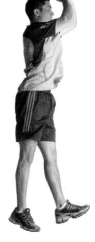

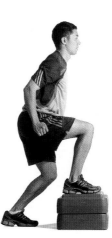
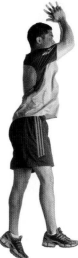

HALF-KNEELING HIGH CABLE STABILITY CHOP

STARTING POSITION:

Half-kneel in an in-line position with your hips perpendicular to a rope-handled high cable pulley machine. Your outside knee should be down, and your inside foot should be on the floor. Hold the rope handle with one hand on the end and the other hand 18 to 24 inches away from it.

PROCEDURE:

Without moving your torso, pull your outside hand to your chest and down. Push your inside hand across your body. Reverse the movement to reach the starting position, and continue for the prescribed number of reps. Then face the opposite direction and repeat with the other arm.

COACHING KEY:

Do not allow any movement throughout your trunk during the exercise. Keep your chest up, your shoulder blades back and down, and your stomach tight. Your feet and knee should be in line.

YOU SHOULD FEEL IT:

Working your shoulders and abdominals.

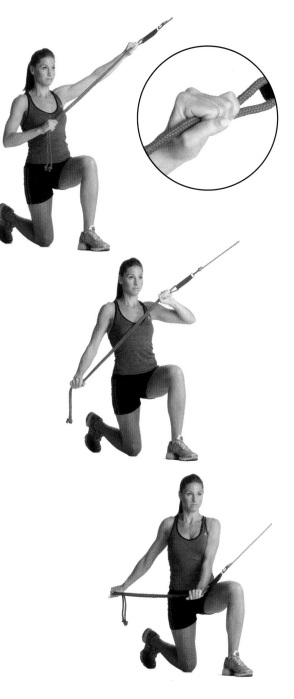

HALF-KNEELING LOW CABLE STABILITY LIFT

STARTING POSITION:

Half-kneel in an in-line position with your hips perpendicular to a low cable pulley machine that has a long rope handle attached. Your inside knee should be down, and your outside foot should be flat on the floor, directly in front of your other knee. Hold the rope handle with one hand on each end.

PROCEDURE:

With your shoulders perpendicular to the machine, your chest up, and your stomach tight, let your arms come in toward the machine, with your outside hand high and your inside hand low. Keeping the rope straight, pull your outside hand diagonally up and across your body to the outside shoulder. Then lift your inside hand straight up to the ceiling. Return to the starting position and repeat. Then face the opposite direction and repeat with the other arm.

COACHING KEY:

Do not let your torso move at all during the movement. Be sure to keep your shoulders perpendicular to the machine. Keep your abs drawn in and your sternum lifted. Your feet and knee should be in line.

YOU SHOULD FEEL IT:

Working your torso rotators and your upper back, chest, and shoulders.

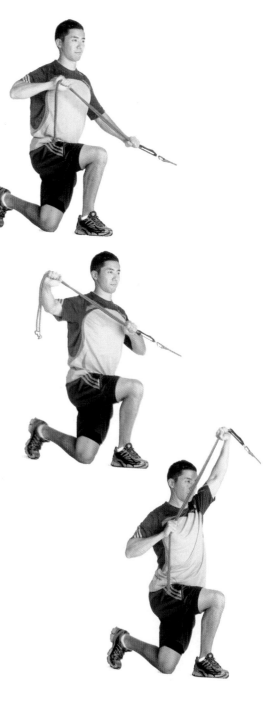

VALSLIDE ECCENTRIC LEG CURL

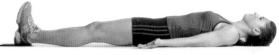

STARTING POSITION:

Lie faceup on the floor, with both heels on Valslides.

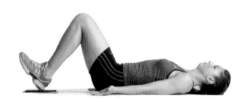

PROCEDURE:

Pull your heels toward your glutes. Lift your hips until your body is in a straight line from knee to shoulder. Keeping your hips extended and off the ground, slowly straighten your legs and then lower your hips to the ground. Repeat for the prescribed number of reps.

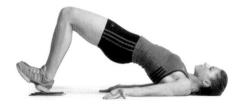

COACHING KEY:

Do not let your hips drop as your heels move away from your glutes. Keep your toes pulled up (see inset).

YOU SHOULD FEEL IT:

Working your glutes, hamstrings, and lower back.

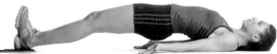

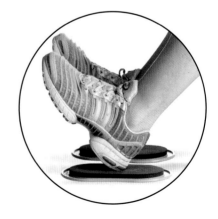

ROMANIAN DEADLIFT TO CABLE ROW

STARTING POSITION:

Stand facing a medium pulley cable station, holding the cable handles with both hands.

PROCEDURE:

Keeping your knees slightly bent and your back flat, hinge over at the hips and reach your arms out in front of you until you feel a mild stretch in your hamstrings. Return to standing position as you pull your elbows back and your forearms slide under your ribs. Continue for the prescribed number of reps.

COACHING KEY:

Keep your back flat and your knees slightly bent throughout the movement. Do not squat during the movement.

YOU SHOULD FEEL IT:

Working your hamstrings, glutes, and back.

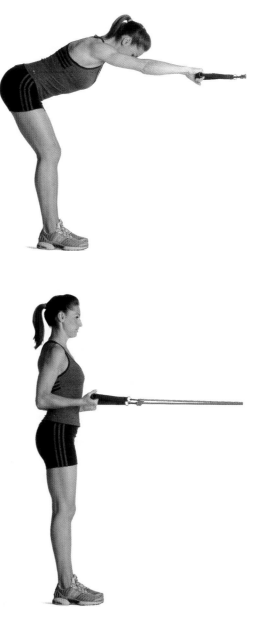

VALSLIDE OR REGULAR SPLIT SQUAT

STARTING POSITION:

Stand with one foot on a Valslide (see inset) or on a slippery surface, such as a file folder on carpeting.

PROCEDURE:

Slide your foot backward and drop your hips to the ground by bending your front knee without letting your back leg touch the ground. Return to the starting position by pushing up with your front leg. Continue for the prescribed number of reps, then switch legs.

COACHING KEY:

Do not let your front knee slide forward past your toes or collapse to the inside. Keep your chest up. Keep the glute of your back leg contracted (tight).

YOU SHOULD FEEL IT:

Working your glutes, hamstrings, and quads, and stretching the hip flexor of your back leg.

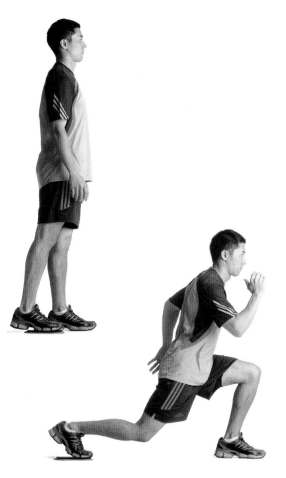

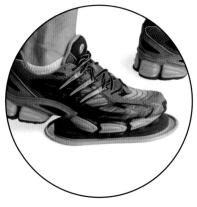

DUMBBELL BENCH PRESS—ALTERNATING

STARTING POSITION:
Lie faceup on a weight bench, holding dumbbells at the outside edges of your shoulders, your palms facing your thighs.

PROCEDURE:
Lift both dumbbells straight up over your chest. Keeping one arm straight, lower the other dumbbell (see inset) until your upper arm is parallel or slightly below parallel to the floor, then push it back up. Then repeat with the other arm. That's 1 repetition.

COACHING KEY:
Make sure to stabilize your extended arm and take the active dumbbell through a full range of motion. Keep your stomach tight so that your trunk does not rotate on the bench as the weight lowers.

YOU SHOULD FEEL IT:
In your chest, shoulders, and triceps.

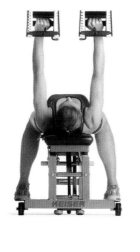

HIGH CABLE SPLIT STABILITY CHOP

STARTING POSITION:

Stand in an in-line scissor position with your hips perpendicular to a rope-handled high cable pulley machine. Your outside leg should be back, and your inside leg should be forward. Hold the rope handle with your inside hand on the end and your outside hand 18 to 24 inches away.

PROCEDURE:

Without moving your torso, pull your outside hand to your chest and down. Push your inside hand across your body. Reverse the movement to the starting position, and continue for the prescribed number of reps. Then face the opposite direction and repeat with the opposite hand inside.

COACHING KEY:

Do not allow any movement throughout your trunk during the exercise. Keep your chest up, your shoulder blades back and down, and your stomach tight.

YOU SHOULD FEEL IT:

Working your shoulders and abs.

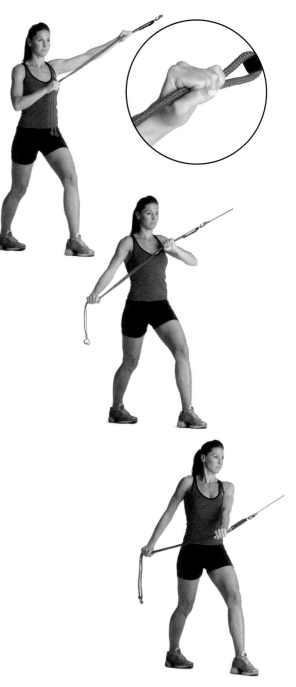

LOW CABLE SPLIT STABILITY LIFT

STARTING POSITION:

Stand in an in-line scissor position with your hips perpendicular a rope-handled low cable pulley machine. Your inside leg should be back, and your outside leg should be forward. Hold the long rope handle with the inside hand on the end and the outside hand 18 to 24 inches apart.

PROCEDURE:

With your shoulders perpendicular to the machine, your chest up, and your stomach tight, let your arms come in toward the machine with your outside hand high and your inside hand low. Keeping the rope straight, diagonally pull your outside hand up and across your body to your outside shoulder. Then lift your inside hand straight up to the ceiling. Return to the starting position and continue for the prescribed number of reps. Then face the opposite direction and repeat with the opposite hand inside.

COACHING KEY:

Do not let your torso move at all during the movement. Be sure to keep your shoulders perpendicular to the machine. Keep your abs drawn in and your sternum lifted.

YOU SHOULD FEEL IT:

Working your torso rotators and your upper back, chest, and shoulders.

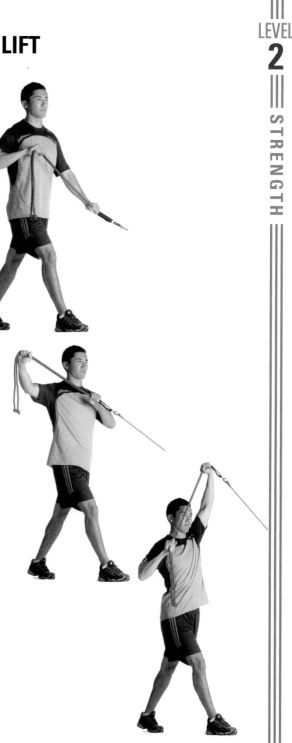

VALSLIDE LEG CURL

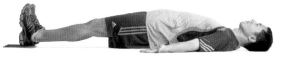

STARTING POSITION:

Lie faceup on the floor, with both heels on the Valslide.

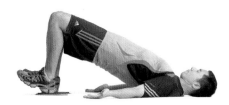

PROCEDURE:

Lift your hips until your body is in a straight line from ankle to shoulder. Keeping your hips tall, pull your heels in toward your glutes. Slowly return to the starting position and continue for the prescribed number of reps.

COACHING KEY:

Do not let your hips drop as your heels come in toward your glutes. Keep your toes pulled up (see inset).

YOU SHOULD FEEL IT:

Working your glutes, hamstrings, and lower back.

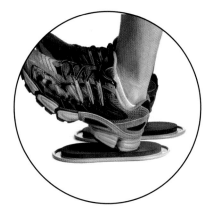

ONE-LEG SQUAT TO CABLE ROW

STARTING POSITION:

Stand on your right leg, facing a medium pulley cable machine. Hold the cable handle in your right hand.

PROCEDURE:

Squat by shifting your hips back and down as you reach forward with your right hand. Then return to the starting position by standing up as you pull your right elbow back and slide your forearm under your ribs. Continue for the prescribed number of reps, then switch legs and arms.

COACHING KEY:

Hold perfect posture. Feel the stretch in your glutes as you squat and accelerate up to vertical running position.

YOU SHOULD FEEL IT:

In your glutes, quads, and upper back.

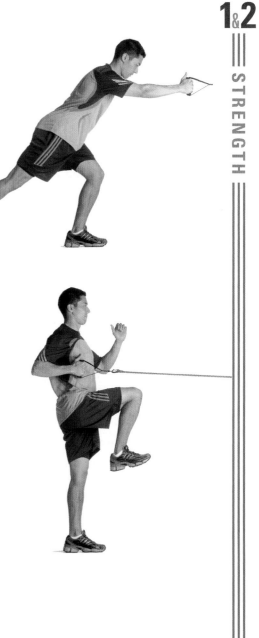

VALSLIDE LATERAL SQUAT

STARTING POSITION:

Stand with one foot on a Valslide (see inset).

PROCEDURE:

Slide your lead foot sideways, keeping your leg straight and the bottom of your foot in contact with the Valslide. As you slide, squat back and down, keeping your weight on the leg that is squatting. Return to the starting position by pushing up with the squatting leg. Continue for the prescribed number of reps, then switch legs.

COACHING KEY:

Keep your toes pointed straight ahead and both feet in full contact with the ground and the Valslide.

YOU SHOULD FEEL IT:

Working your glutes, hamstrings, and quads, and stretching the groin area of your straight leg.

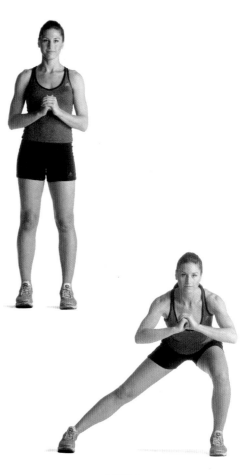

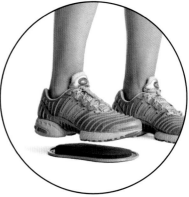

VALSLIDE PUSHUP

STARTING POSITION:

Assume a pushup position with each hand on a Valslide (see inset).

PROCEDURE:

With your belly button drawn in, lower yourself to where your chest is 4 to 6 inches off the floor. Control as you push back up, holding your belly button in and pushing your sternum as far away from the floor as possible. Continue for the prescribed number of reps.

COACHING KEY:

Keep your body straight from ear to ankle.

YOU SHOULD FEEL IT:

Working your chest, shoulders, and arms.

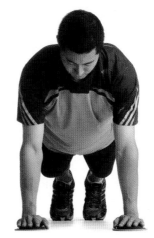

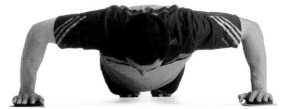

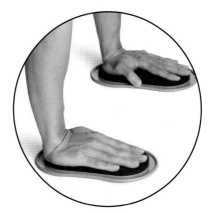

DUMBBELL BENCH PRESS

STARTING POSITION:

Lie faceup on a weight bench, holding dumb-bells over your shoulders, your palms facing your thighs.

PROCEDURE:

Lift both dumbbells straight up over your chest. Lower both dumbbells until your upper arms are parallel to the ground, then push them back up. That's 1 repetition.

COACHING KEY:

Keep your stomach tight through the move-ment. Do not let your back arch as you press the dumbbells up.

YOU SHOULD FEEL IT:

In your chest, shoulders, and triceps.

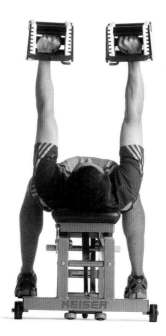

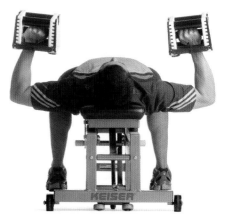

FOAM ROLL EXERCISES

Using a foam roll is the next best thing to getting a professional massage. By using one on the areas as described on the following pages, you'll find that you get much of the benefit, without the cost of a massage therapist.

The more uncomfortable a muscle feels during the foam roll treatment, the more it needs to be massaged. Hold on sore spots for an extended time (30 to 90 seconds) to release them before moving on to the next sore spot.

CALF

STARTING POSITION:

Sit on the ground with your legs straight, your left leg crossed over the right, and a foam roll under your right calf.

PROCEDURE:

Lift your butt off the ground so that your weight is supported by your hands and the foam roll only. Roll the length of your calf, from your Achilles to behind your knee, and repeat for 30 to 60 seconds per leg.

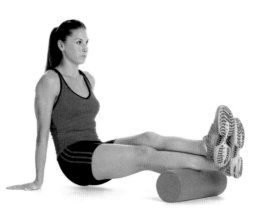

COACHING KEY:

Place as much weight as possible on the roll Hold on sore spots for 30 to 60 seconds.

YOU SHOULD FEEL:

As if you were getting a deep massage.

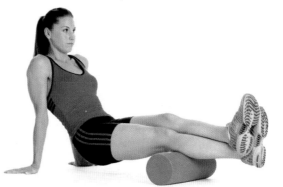

PERONEALS

STARTING POSITION:

Lie on your side with your knees pulled to your chest and a foam roll under the side of your lower leg. Your weight should be supported on the roll and your elbow.

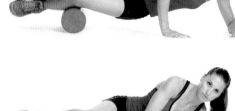

PROCEDURE:

Roll the length of your lower leg, from just below the outside of your knee down to your ankle. Repeat for 30 to 60 seconds per leg.

COACHING KEY:

Place as much weight as possible on the roll. Hold on sore spots for 30 to 60 seconds.

YOU SHOULD FEEL:

As if you were getting a deep massage.

TIBIALIS ANTERIOR

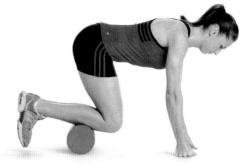

STARTING POSITION:

Get on your hands and knees with a foam roll under the front of your shins, just below your knees.

PROCEDURE:

Keeping your hands still, roll your knees toward your hands, rolling the front of your shins from just below your knees to your ankles. Repeat for 30 to 60 seconds.

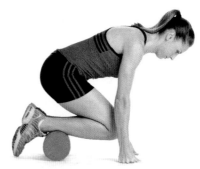

COACHING KEY:

Keep your back flat and stomach tight throughout the movement. Place as much weight as possible on the roll. Hold on sore spots for 30 to 60 seconds.

YOU SHOULD FEEL:

As if you were getting a deep massage.

HAMSTRING

STARTING POSITION:

Sit on the ground with a foam roll under the back of one thigh and other leg crossed over it.

PROCEDURE:

Roll over the foam, moving it up and down the length of the back of your thigh, for 30 to 60 seconds. Then switch legs and repeat.

COACHING KEY:

If the massage feels too sensitive, uncross your legs and roll both hamstrings at once. Hold on sore spots for 30 to 60 seconds.

YOU SHOULD FEEL:

As if you were getting a deep massage.

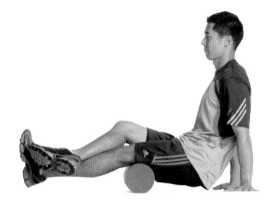

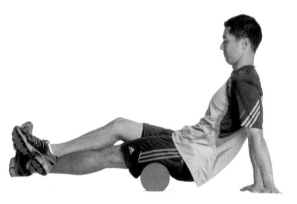

QUAD/HIP FLEXOR

STARTING POSITION:

Lie facedown on the ground with a foam roll under one thigh, with the other leg crossed at the ankles.

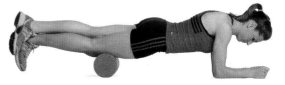

PROCEDURE:

Roll along the quads from your hip to just above your knees for 30 to 60 seconds per leg.

COACHING KEY:

For added benefit, roll slightly on the outside and inside as well as down the front of the thigh. Hold on sore spots for 30 to 60 seconds.

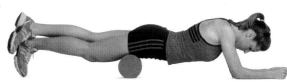

YOU SHOULD FEEL:

As if you were getting a deep massage.

VMO (VASTUS MEDIALIS OBLIQUUS)

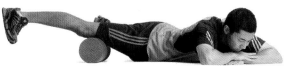

STARTING POSITION:

Lie facedown on the ground with one leg to the side, the foam roll just above the inside of your knee.

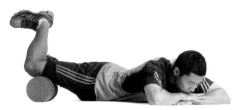

PROCEDURE:

Slowly bend and straighten your leg 10 times. Adjust the roll to find a new sore spot and repeat.

COACHING KEY:

Hold on sore spots for 30 to 60 seconds.

YOU SHOULD FEEL:

As if you were getting a deep massage.

ADDUCTOR

STARTING POSITION:

Lie facedown on the ground with one leg to the side and a foam roll under the inside of your other thigh.

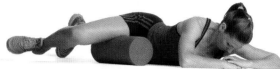

PROCEDURE:

Roll along the inside of your thigh from your pelvis to the inside of your knee for 30 to 60 seconds. Then switch legs and repeat.

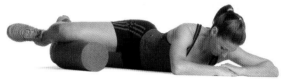

COACHING KEY:

Hold on sore spots for 30 to 60 seconds.

YOU SHOULD FEEL:

As if you were getting a deep massage.

TFL (TENSOR FASCIAE LATAE)

STARTING POSITION:

Lie facedown with a foam roll under your hip.

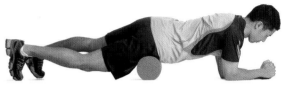

PROCEDURE:

Roll the muscle on the front and slightly to the outside of your upper thigh just below the pelvis for 30 to 60 seconds per leg.

COACHING KEY:

Hold on sore spots for 30 to 60 seconds.

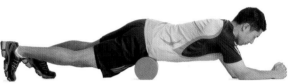

YOU SHOULD FEEL:

As if you were getting a deep massage.

LOWER BACK AND QL (QUADRATUS LUMBORUM)

STARTING POSITION:

Lie faceup on the ground, with a foam roll under the outside of your mid-back, just below your rib cage.

PROCEDURE:

Roll from the middle of your back down to your pelvis and repeat for 30 to 60 seconds per side.

COACHING KEY:

Hold on sore spots for 30 to 60 seconds.

YOU SHOULD FEEL:

As if you were getting a deep massage.

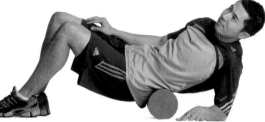

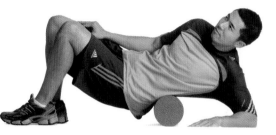

MID- AND UPPER BACK

STARTING POSITION:

Lie faceup on the ground, with a foam roll under your mid-back and your head supported with your hands. Keep your elbows together.

PROCEDURE:

Roll from your shoulders down to the middle of your back and repeat for 30 to 60 seconds.

COACHING KEY:

Hold your hands behind your head with your elbows pointed to the sky and close together. Hold on sore spots for 30 to 60 seconds.

YOU SHOULD FEEL:

As if you were getting a deep massage.

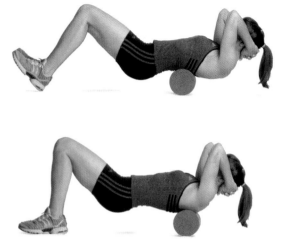

LAT (LATISSIMUS DORSI)

STARTING POSITION:

Lie on your side on the ground, with a foam roll under your lower back.

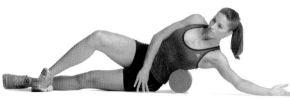

PROCEDURE:

Roll from the side of your lower back up to your armpit for 30 to 60 seconds. Then switch sides and repeat.

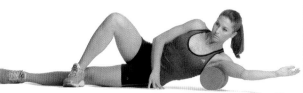

COACHING KEY:

Hold on sore spots for 30 to 60 seconds.

YOU SHOULD FEEL:

As if you were getting a deep massage.

REGENERATION

AIS (ACTIVE-ISOLATED STRETCHING)—GASTROCNEMIUS (CALF)

STARTING POSITION:

Lie on your back with a rope wrapped around your right foot and your leg raised 45 degrees into the air.

PROCEDURE:

Actively pull your right foot to your shin and then give assistance with the rope. Hold the stretch for 1 to 2 seconds and then relax. Perform 10 times then switch legs.

COACHING KEY:

Exhale during the stretch. Continue to actively pull your foot to your shin even when assisting with the rope.

YOU SHOULD FEEL IT:

Stretching your calf.

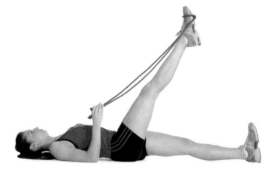

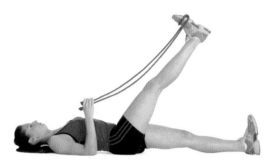

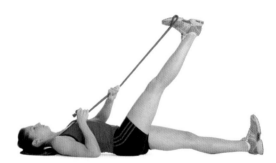

AIS—SOLEUS

STARTING POSITION:

Sit with your right leg in front of your body with your knee bent.

PROCEDURE:

Actively pull your right foot to your shin. Grabbing the foot with both hands, pull the foot farther to the shin until you feel a stretch in your calf and Achilles. Hold the stretch for 1 to 2 seconds and then relax. Perform 10 times then switch legs.

COACHING KEY:

Exhale during the stretch. Continue to actively pull your foot to your shin even when pulling with your hands.

YOU SHOULD FEEL IT:

Stretching your calf and Achilles.

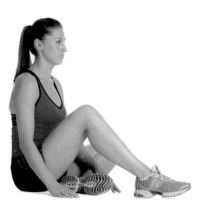

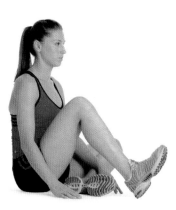

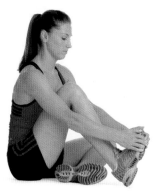

AIS—BENT-LEG HAMSTRING

STARTING POSITION:

Lie on your back with your right knee pulled to your chest and a rope wrapped around your right foot.

PROCEDURE:

Actively straighten the right knee as much as possible without letting it move away from your chest. Give gentle assistance with the rope until you feel a stretch, hold 2 seconds, and relax. Continue for 10 repetitions, then switch legs and repeat.

COACHING KEY:

Keep your opposite leg on the ground by pushing your heel as far away from your head as possible, contracting your glute. Keep your knee pulled as tightly to your chest as possible throughout entire movement. Pull your rope above head. It's okay if you can't fully straighten your knee.

YOU SHOULD FEEL:

Stretching in the hamstring of the bent leg, and stretching in the hip flexor of the bottom leg.

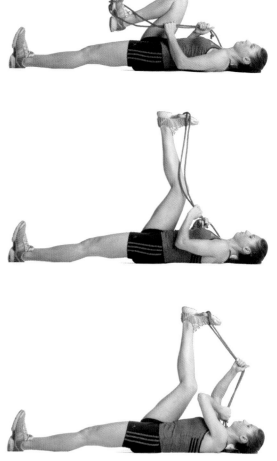

AIS—STRAIGHT-LEG HAMSTRING

STARTING POSITION:

Lie on your back with your right leg straight and a rope wrapped around your foot.

PROCEDURE:

Keeping your right leg straight, actively lift it as high as possible, then give gentle assistance with the rope until you feel a stretch. Hold 2 seconds and relax. Repeat for 10 repetitions, then switch legs.

COACHING KEY:

Keep your opposite leg on the ground by pushing your heel as far away from your head as possible, contracting the glute. Pull the rope above your head.

YOU SHOULD FEEL:

Stretching in the hamstring of the raised leg, and stretching in the hip flexor of the bottom leg.

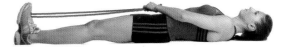

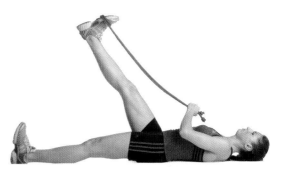

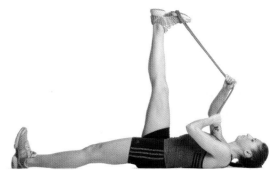

AIS—KNEELING QUAD/HIP FLEXOR

STARTING POSITION:

Half-kneel (put one knee on the ground) with your back knee on a soft mat or pad. Rest the hand of your opposite arm on your forward knee.

PROCEDURE:

While keeping a slight forward lean in your torso, tighten your stomach and contract the glute of your back leg. Maintaining this posture, shift your entire body slightly forward. Exhale and hold the stretch for 2 seconds. Relax, repeat 10 times, and then switch legs.

COACHING KEY:

Avoid excessive arching in your lower back.

YOU SHOULD FEEL:

Stretching in the front of your hip and upper thigh of your back leg.

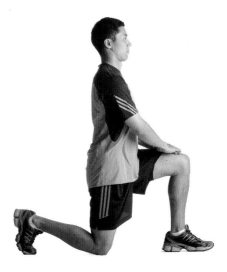

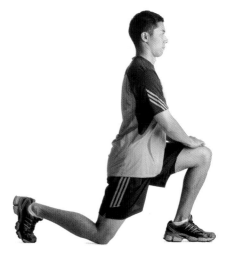

AIS—ABDUCTOR

STARTING POSITION:

Lie on your back with a rope wrapped around the outside of one foot (see inset). Hold the end of the rope in your opposite hand, with your free hand out to the side.

PROCEDURE:

Actively lift your leg across your body as far as possible, and then give gentle assistance with the rope until you feel a stretch. Exhale and hold for 2 seconds, then relax and repeat for 10 repetitions. Then switch legs.

COACHING KEY:

Keep your non-roped leg on the ground by pushing your heel as far away from your head as possible, contracting the glute. Keep your toes pointed to the sky. Keep your back in line and your shoulders on the ground.

YOU SHOULD FEEL:

Stretching in the outside of the thigh of your roped leg.

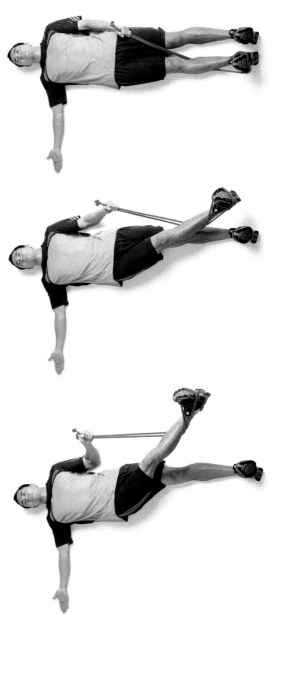

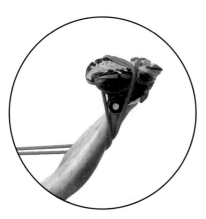

AIS—ADDUCTOR

STARTING POSITION:

Lie on your back with a rope wrapped around one foot. The rope should be wrapped around the inside of your lower leg (see inset). Hold the end of the rope in the hand on the same side as your roped leg.

PROCEDURE:

Actively lift your leg as far to the side as possible, then give gentle assistance with the rope until you feel a stretch. Exhale and hold for 2 seconds, then relax and repeat for 10 repetitions. Then switch sides.

COACHING KEY:

Keep your opposite leg on the ground by pushing your heel as far away from your head as possible, contracting the glute. Keep your toes pointed to the sky. Keep your back in line and your shoulders on the ground.

YOU SHOULD FEEL:

Stretching in the inside of the thigh of the leg with the rope.

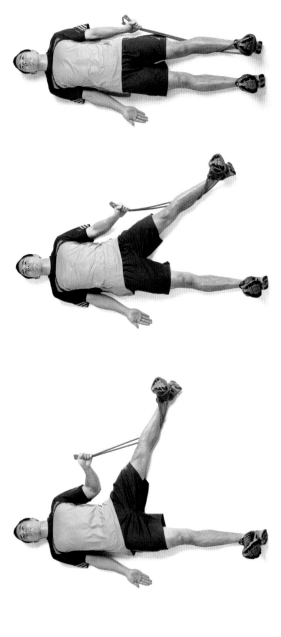

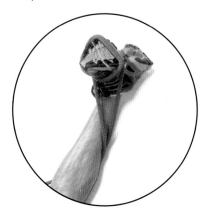

AIS—CHEST STRETCH

STARTING POSITION:

Assume a stride stance with your arms in front of your body and your palms up.

PROCEDURE:

Keeping your stomach tight and your back glute contracted, reach both arms behind you until you feel a gentle stretch in your chest and arms. Hold for 2 seconds and return to the starting position. Repeat for 5 repetitions, then switch legs.

COACHING KEY:

Maintain perfect posture.

YOU SHOULD FEEL:

Stretching in your chest.

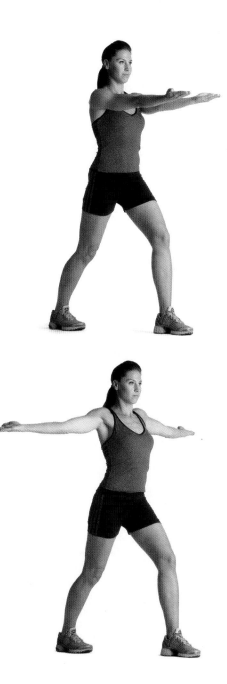

AIS—SHOULDER (SIDE LYING)

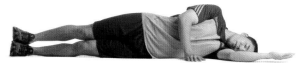

STARTING POSITION:

Lie on your side with the upper part of your bottom arm parallel to your belt line and your elbow bent 90 degrees.

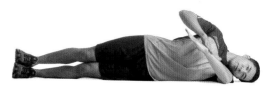

PROCEDURE:

Rotate the palm of your bottom toward the ground as far as possible, gently pressing your palm farther with the other hand. Hold 2 seconds, relax, and repeat 10 times. Then switch sides.

COACHING KEY:

Actively try to rotate your palm toward the ground throughout the entire movement. Keep your chin tucked and do not let your bottom shoulder rise off the ground. Start with a small range of motion and gradually increase it.

YOU SHOULD FEEL:

Stretching in your back and the inside of your bottom shoulder.

ROPE TRICEPS/SHOULDER STRETCH

STARTING POSITION:

Stand holding a rope behind your head with your right hand over and your left hand under.

PROCEDURE:

Actively reach your right hand down your back and give gentle assistance with your left hand, exhaling and holding the stretch for 2 seconds. Now, actively reach your left hand up your back as high as possible, and give gentle assistance with your right hand, exhaling and holding the stretch for 2 seconds. Repeat for 10 repetitions, then switch hands and repeat.

COACHING KEY:

Actively move through the range of motion with the arm being stretched. Exhale during the stretch. Maintain perfect posture with your stomach tightened.

YOU SHOULD FEEL:

Stretching in the triceps of the top arm, and stretching in the shoulder of the bottom arm.

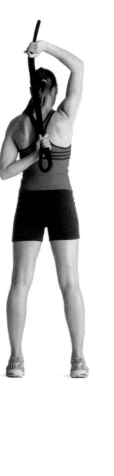

FOAM ROLL STRETCH—REACH, ROLL, AND LIFT

STARTING POSITION:

Sit on your heels with your arms extended and the backs of your hands on a foam roll.

PROCEDURE:

Roll the foam forward while keeping your hips back and your chest dropped toward the floor. Lift and exhale as you hold the stretch for 2 seconds. Return to the starting position and repeat.

COACHING KEY:

Attempt to lift your hands off the foam roll as you exhale, but keep your hands in contact with the foam.

YOU SHOULD FEEL:

Stretching in your upper back and shoulders.

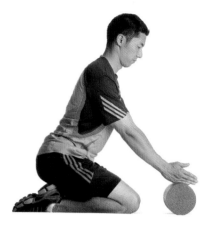

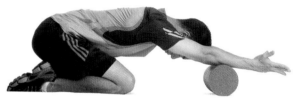

ARCH ROLL

STARTING POSITION:

Stand with your shoes off.

PROCEDURE:

Place one foot on a tennis ball. Roll the arch of your foot back and forth over the ball 50 times. Hold on any trigger point for 30 to 90 seconds. Then switch feet and repeat.

COACHING KEY:

The more uncomfortable it is, the more the muscle needs to be massaged. Hold on sore spots for an extended time to release them. Roll through different angles to cover the entire arch of your foot.

YOU SHOULD FEEL:

As if you were getting a deep massage on the bottom of your foot.

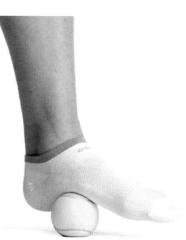

REGENERATION

PEC MINOR

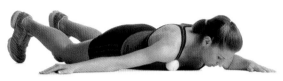

STARTING POSITION:

Lie on your stomach with a tennis ball under one of your pectoral (upper chest) muscles (see inset).

PROCEDURE:

Adjust your position on the ball until you find a sore trigger point. Hold on the spot for 60 to 90 seconds. Then switch pectorals and repeat.

COACHING KEY:

Try to maintain as much body weight on the ball as possible. The more painful it is, the more your muscle needs to be massaged.

YOU SHOULD FEEL:

As if you were getting a deep massage to your chest.

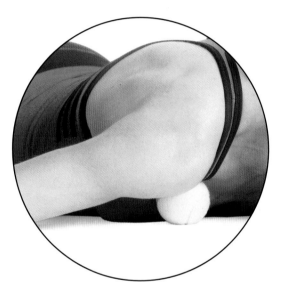

IT (ILIOTIBIAL) BAND WITH TENNIS BALL

STARTING POSITION:

Lie on your side with a tennis ball under the outside of your upper thigh.

PROCEDURE:

Adjust your position on the ball until you find a sore trigger point. Hold on the spot for 60 to 90 seconds. Move the ball halfway down your thigh and repeat. Then move the ball just above your knee (see inset) and repeat.

COACHING KEY:

Try to maintain as much body weight on the ball as possible. The more painful it is, the more your muscle needs to be massaged.

YOU SHOULD FEEL:

As if you were getting a deep massage to the outside of your thigh.

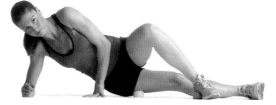

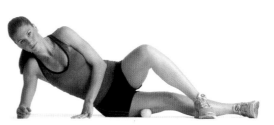

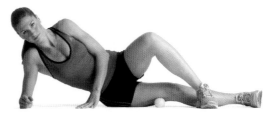

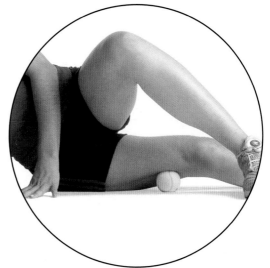

PIRIFORMIS

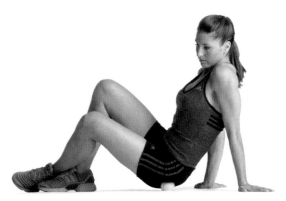

STARTING POSITION:

Sit on one hip with a tennis ball under the outside of one of your glutes (see inset).

PROCEDURE:

Adjust your position on the ball until you find a sore trigger point. Hold on the spot for 60 to 90 seconds. Move the ball to a slightly different spot and repeat.

COACHING KEY:

Try to maintain as much body weight on the ball as possible. The more painful it is, the more your muscle needs to be massaged. If you experience numbness or tingling in your foot, adjust the ball to a different spot.

YOU SHOULD FEEL:

As if you were getting a deep massage to your glute and piriformis (a muscle in your hip rotator complex).

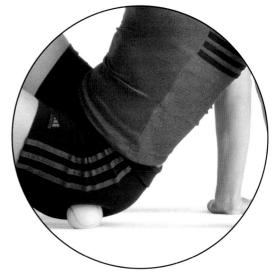

VMO (VASTUS MEDIALIS OBLIQUUS) WITH TENNIS BALL

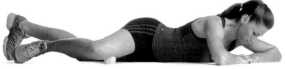

STARTING POSITION:

Lie on your stomach with a tennis ball just above your knee (see inset).

PROCEDURE:

Adjust your position on the ball until you find a sore trigger point. Hold on the spot for 60 to 90 seconds.

COACHING KEY:

Try to maintain as much body weight on the ball as possible. The more painful it is, the more your muscle needs to be massaged.

YOU SHOULD FEEL:

As if you were getting a deep massage to your VMO.

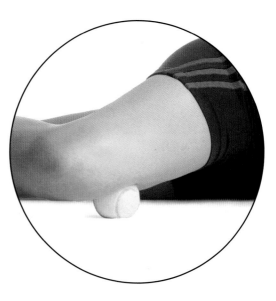

THORACIC SPINE

STARTING POSITION:

Tape two tennis balls together to form a "peanut" shape (see inset). Lie on your back with the balls under your spine just above your lower back and your hands behind your head.

PROCEDURE:

Perform 5 crunches, then raise your arms over your chest, and alternately reach over your head for 5 repetitions with each arm. Move the ball up your spine 1 to 2 inches and repeat the crunches and arm reaches. Continue moving up your spine until you are just above your shoulder blades and below the base of your neck.

COACHING KEY:

During the crunches, try to "hinge" on the ball rather than rolling over it. Think about keeping your ribs pushed down to the floor during the arm reaches.

YOU SHOULD FEEL:

As if you were getting a deep massage in your mid- to upper back.

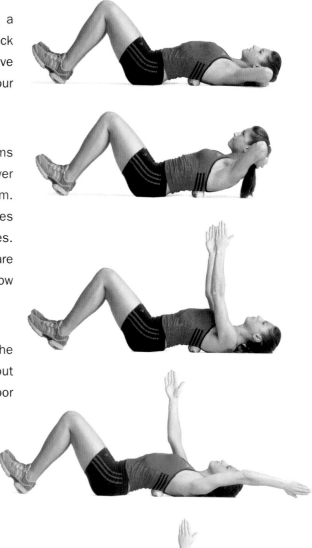

Here's an at-a-glance look at your Core Performance calendar. In the basic program, you'll alternate weeks, depending on what week of the month it is. You'll follow the Odd Weeks schedule on the 1st, 3rd, and (if applicable) 5th weeks of the month, and the Even Weeks schedule on the 2nd and 4th weeks. Note that the days aren't labeled Sunday through Saturday or Monday through Sunday. This is intentional, recognizing that not everyone takes the same day off. If Thursday is your day off, for example, count Friday as day 2.

The race week program begins with "Race Day −5," which is simply the 5th day out from the event. "Race Day +1" is the day after the event. We recommend going through Levels 1 and 2 in the basic program before progressing to the advanced program.

Even though you have specific regeneration days, it's always recommended to incorporate some Regeneration strategies post-workout on your power and strength days. Feel free to pick and choose from the exercises on pages 208 to 213, based on your needs, but save the Energy System Development (ESD) work for specific regeneration days.

BASIC PROGRAM

ODD WEEKS

DAY 1	DAY 2	DAY 3	DAY 4	DAY 5	DAY 6	DAY 7
Off	Power	Regeneration	Strength	Regeneration	Power	Regeneration

EVEN WEEKS

DAY 1	DAY 2	DAY 3	DAY 4	DAY 5	DAY 6	DAY 7
Off	Strength	Regeneration	Power	Regeneration	Strength	Regeneration

ADVANCED PROGRAM

DAY 1	DAY 2	DAY 3	DAY 4	DAY 5	DAY 6	DAY 7
Off	Power	Strength	Regeneration	Power	Strength	Regeneration

RACE WEEK

RACE DAY−5	RACE DAY −4	RACE DAY −3	RACE DAY −2	RACE DAY −1	RACE DAY	RACE DAY +1
Strength	Regeneration	Power	Regeneration	Regeneration	Movement Prep	Regeneration

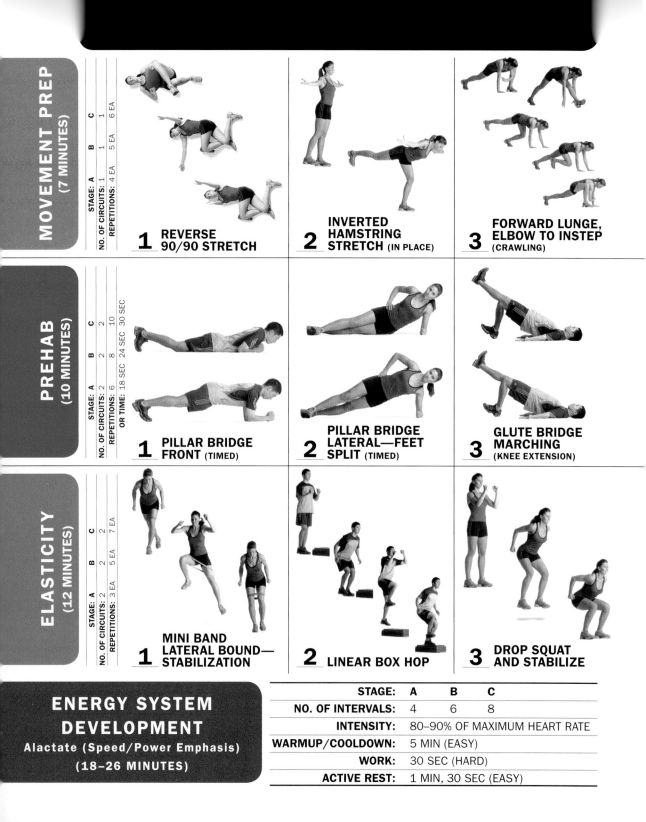

MOVEMENT PREP (7 MINUTES)

	STAGE:	A	B	C
	NO. OF CIRCUITS:	1	1	1
	REPETITIONS:	4 EA	5 EA	6 EA

1 REVERSE 90/90 STRETCH

2 INVERTED HAMSTRING STRETCH (IN PLACE)

3 FORWARD LUNGE, ELBOW TO INSTEP (CRAWLING)

PREHAB (10 MINUTES)

	STAGE:	A	B	C
	NO. OF CIRCUITS:	2	2	2
	REPETITIONS:	6	8	10
	OR TIME:	18 SEC	24 SEC	30 SEC

1 PILLAR BRIDGE FRONT (TIMED)

2 PILLAR BRIDGE LATERAL—FEET SPLIT (TIMED)

3 GLUTE BRIDGE MARCHING (KNEE EXTENSION)

ELASTICITY (12 MINUTES)

	STAGE:	A	B	C
	NO. OF CIRCUITS:	2	2	2
	REPETITIONS:	3 EA	5 EA	7 EA

1 MINI BAND LATERAL BOUND— STABILIZATION

2 LINEAR BOX HOP

3 DROP SQUAT AND STABILIZE

ENERGY SYSTEM DEVELOPMENT
Alactate (Speed/Power Emphasis)
(18–26 MINUTES)

	STAGE:	A	B	C
NO. OF INTERVALS:		4	6	8
INTENSITY:		80–90% OF MAXIMUM HEART RATE		
WARMUP/COOLDOWN:		5 MIN (EASY)		
WORK:		30 SEC (HARD)		
ACTIVE REST:		1 MIN, 30 SEC (EASY)		

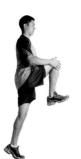

4 KNEE HUG (IN PLACE)

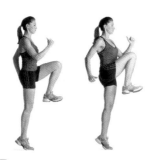

5 PILLAR MARCH (MOVING)

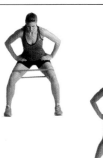

4 MINI BAND INTERNAL/
EXTERNAL ROTATION

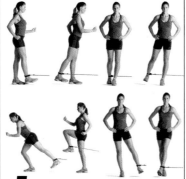

5 FOUR-WAY HIP CABLE

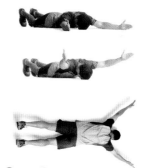

6 FLOOR Ys

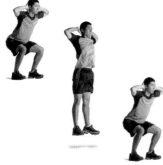

4 SQUAT JUMP—NON-
COUNTERMOVEMENT

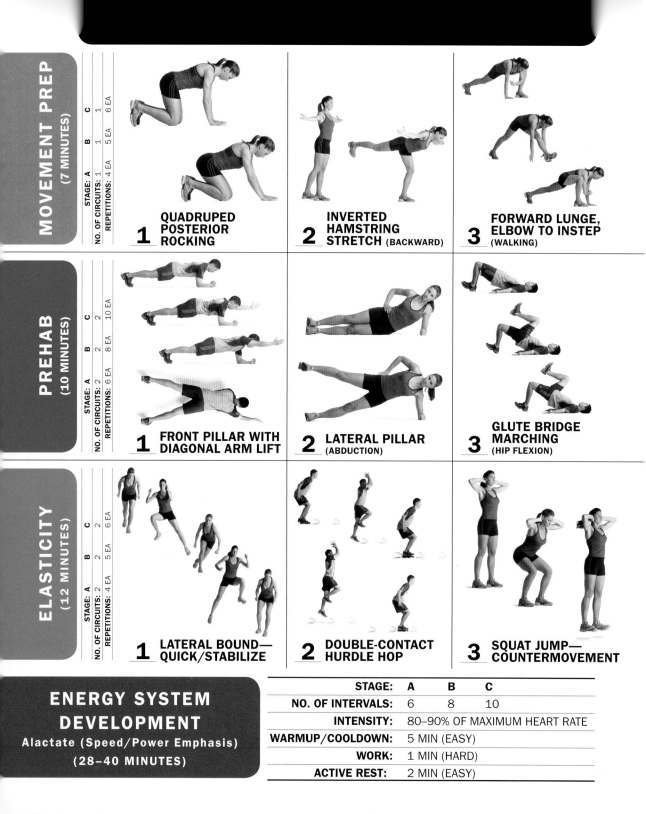

MOVEMENT PREP (7 MINUTES)

STAGE:	A	B	C
NO. OF CIRCUITS:	1	1	1
REPETITIONS:	4 EA	5 EA	6 EA

1 QUADRUPED POSTERIOR ROCKING

2 INVERTED HAMSTRING STRETCH (BACKWARD)

3 FORWARD LUNGE, ELBOW TO INSTEP (WALKING)

PREHAB (10 MINUTES)

STAGE:	A	B	C
NO. OF CIRCUITS:	2	2	2
REPETITIONS:	6 EA	8 EA	10 EA

1 FRONT PILLAR WITH DIAGONAL ARM LIFT

2 LATERAL PILLAR (ABDUCTION)

3 GLUTE BRIDGE MARCHING (HIP FLEXION)

ELASTICITY (12 MINUTES)

STAGE:	A	B	C
NO. OF CIRCUITS:	2	2	2
REPETITIONS:	4 EA	5 EA	6 EA

1 LATERAL BOUND— QUICK/STABILIZE

2 DOUBLE-CONTACT HURDLE HOP

3 SQUAT JUMP— COUNTERMOVEMENT

ENERGY SYSTEM DEVELOPMENT
Alactate (Speed/Power Emphasis)
(28–40 MINUTES)

	STAGE:	A	B	C
	NO. OF INTERVALS:	6	8	10
	INTENSITY:	80–90% OF MAXIMUM HEART RATE		
	WARMUP/COOLDOWN:	5 MIN (EASY)		
	WORK:	1 MIN (HARD)		
	ACTIVE REST:	2 MIN (EASY)		

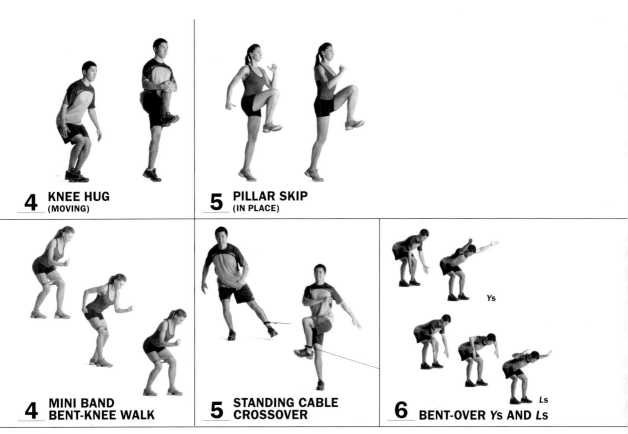

4 KNEE HUG
(MOVING)

5 PILLAR SKIP
(IN PLACE)

4 MINI BAND
BENT-KNEE WALK

5 STANDING CABLE
CROSSOVER

6 BENT-OVER Ys AND Ls

Ys

Ls

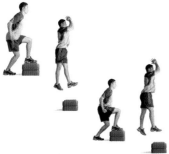

4 REACTIVE STEPUP

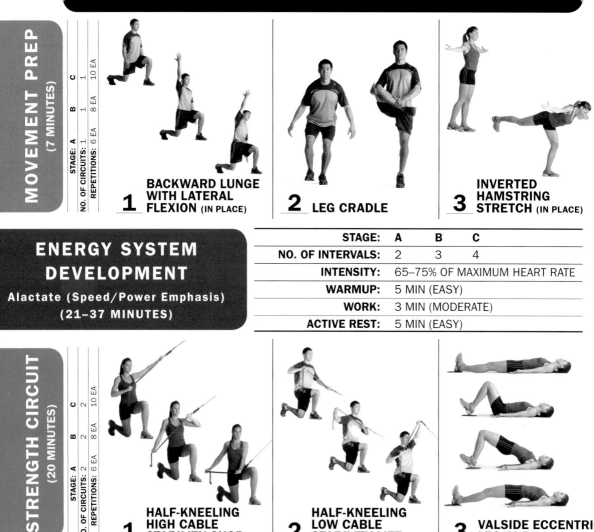

MOVEMENT PREP
(7 MINUTES)

STAGE:	A	B	C
NO. OF CIRCUITS:	1	1	1
REPETITIONS:	6 EA	8 EA	10 EA

1 BACKWARD LUNGE WITH LATERAL FLEXION (IN PLACE)

2 LEG CRADLE

3 INVERTED HAMSTRING STRETCH (IN PLACE)

ENERGY SYSTEM DEVELOPMENT
Alactate (Speed/Power Emphasis)
(21–37 MINUTES)

STAGE:	A	B	C
NO. OF INTERVALS:	2	3	4
INTENSITY:	65–75% OF MAXIMUM HEART RATE		
WARMUP:	5 MIN (EASY)		
WORK:	3 MIN (MODERATE)		
ACTIVE REST:	5 MIN (EASY)		

STRENGTH CIRCUIT
(20 MINUTES)

STAGE:	A	B	C
NO. OF CIRCUITS:	2	2	2
REPETITIONS:	6 EA	8 EA	10 EA

1 HALF-KNEELING HIGH CABLE STABILITY CHOP

2 HALF-KNEELING LOW CABLE STABILITY LIFT

3 VALSIDE ECCENTRIC LEG CURL

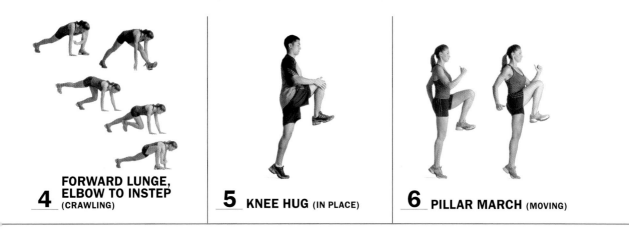

4 **FORWARD LUNGE, ELBOW TO INSTEP** (CRAWLING)

5 **KNEE HUG** (IN PLACE)

6 **PILLAR MARCH** (MOVING)

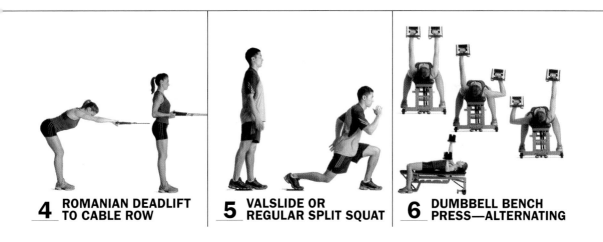

4 **ROMANIAN DEADLIFT TO CABLE ROW**

5 **VALSLIDE OR REGULAR SPLIT SQUAT**

6 **DUMBBELL BENCH PRESS—ALTERNATING**

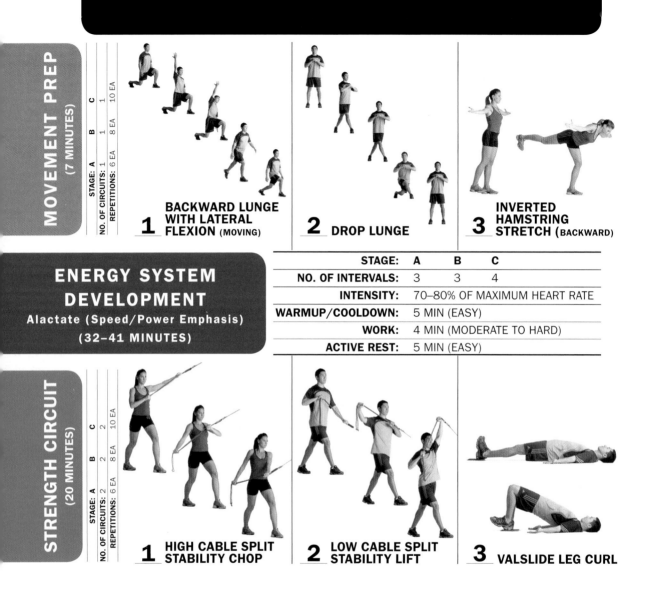

MOVEMENT PREP (7 MINUTES)

	STAGE: A	B	C
NO. OF CIRCUITS:	1	1	1
REPETITIONS:	6 EA	8 EA	10 EA

1 BACKWARD LUNGE WITH LATERAL FLEXION (MOVING)

2 DROP LUNGE

3 INVERTED HAMSTRING STRETCH (BACKWARD)

ENERGY SYSTEM DEVELOPMENT
Alactate (Speed/Power Emphasis)
(32–41 MINUTES)

	STAGE:	A	B	C
	NO. OF INTERVALS:	3	3	4
	INTENSITY:	70–80% OF MAXIMUM HEART RATE		
	WARMUP/COOLDOWN:	5 MIN (EASY)		
	WORK:	4 MIN (MODERATE TO HARD)		
	ACTIVE REST:	5 MIN (EASY)		

STRENGTH CIRCUIT (20 MINUTES)

	STAGE: A	B	C
NO. OF CIRCUITS:	2	2	2
REPETITIONS:	6 EA	8 EA	10 EA

1 HIGH CABLE SPLIT STABILITY CHOP

2 LOW CABLE SPLIT STABILITY LIFT

3 VALSLIDE LEG CURL

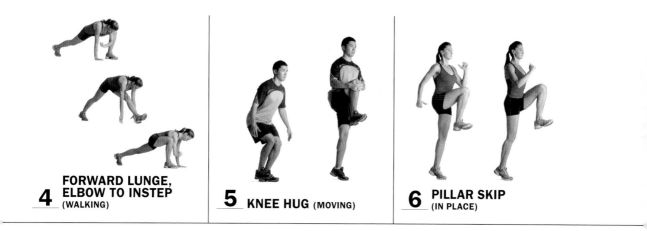

4 **FORWARD LUNGE, ELBOW TO INSTEP** (WALKING)

5 **KNEE HUG** (MOVING)

6 **PILLAR SKIP** (IN PLACE)

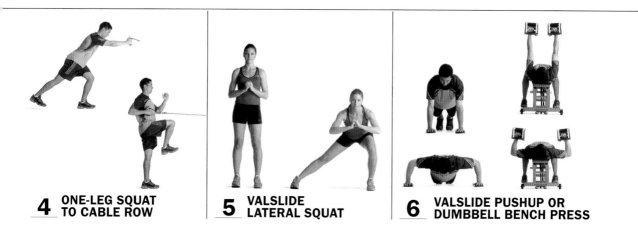

4 **ONE-LEG SQUAT TO CABLE ROW**

5 **VALSLIDE LATERAL SQUAT**

6 **VALSLIDE PUSHUP OR DUMBBELL BENCH PRESS**

REGENERATION DAY WORKOUTS

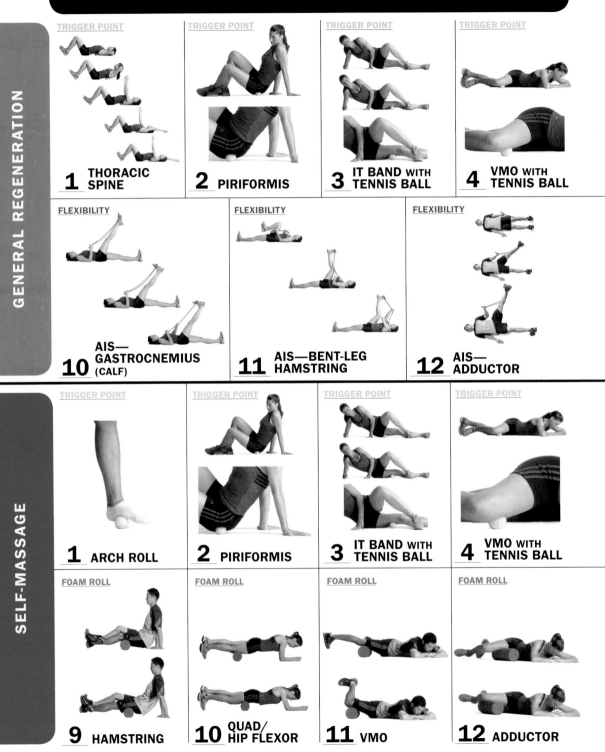

GENERAL REGENERATION

TRIGGER POINT
1 THORACIC SPINE

TRIGGER POINT
2 PIRIFORMIS

TRIGGER POINT
3 IT BAND WITH TENNIS BALL

TRIGGER POINT
4 VMO WITH TENNIS BALL

FLEXIBILITY
10 AIS— GASTROCNEMIUS (CALF)

FLEXIBILITY
11 AIS—BENT-LEG HAMSTRING

FLEXIBILITY
12 AIS— ADDUCTOR

SELF-MASSAGE

TRIGGER POINT
1 ARCH ROLL

TRIGGER POINT
2 PIRIFORMIS

TRIGGER POINT
3 IT BAND WITH TENNIS BALL

TRIGGER POINT
4 VMO WITH TENNIS BALL

FOAM ROLL
9 HAMSTRING

FOAM ROLL
10 QUAD/ HIP FLEXOR

FOAM ROLL
11 VMO

FOAM ROLL
12 ADDUCTOR

ENERGY SYSTEM DEVELOPMENT
Aerobic (Recovery Emphasis)

LEVEL 1 (20–40+ MINUTES)

	STAGE:	A	B	C
	TOTAL TIME:	20 MIN	30 MIN	40+ MIN
	INTENSITY:	60–65% OF MAXIMUM HEART RATE		

LEVEL 2 (30–50+ MINUTES)

	STAGE:	A	B	C
	TOTAL TIME:	30 MIN	40 MIN	50+ MIN
	INTENSITY:	60–65% OF MAXIMUM HEART RATE		

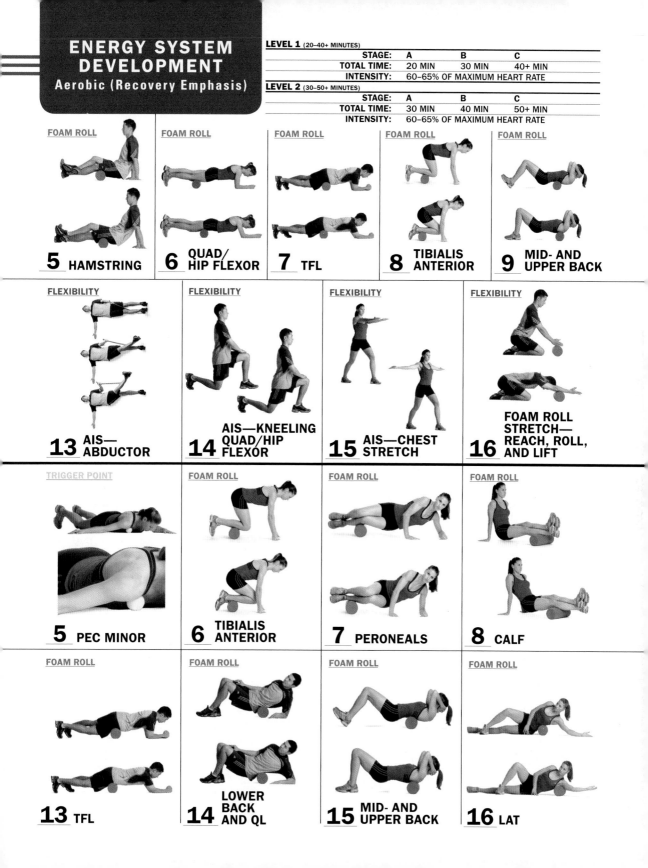

FOAM ROLL

5 HAMSTRING

FOAM ROLL

6 QUAD/ HIP FLEXOR

FOAM ROLL

7 TFL

FOAM ROLL

8 TIBIALIS ANTERIOR

FOAM ROLL

9 MID- AND UPPER BACK

FLEXIBILITY

13 AIS— ABDUCTOR

FLEXIBILITY

14 AIS—KNEELING QUAD/HIP FLEXOR

FLEXIBILITY

15 AIS—CHEST STRETCH

FLEXIBILITY

16 FOAM ROLL STRETCH— REACH, ROLL, AND LIFT

TRIGGER POINT

5 PEC MINOR

FOAM ROLL

6 TIBIALIS ANTERIOR

FOAM ROLL

7 PERONEALS

FOAM ROLL

8 CALF

FOAM ROLL

13 TFL

FOAM ROLL

14 LOWER BACK AND QL

FOAM ROLL

15 MID- AND UPPER BACK

FOAM ROLL

16 LAT

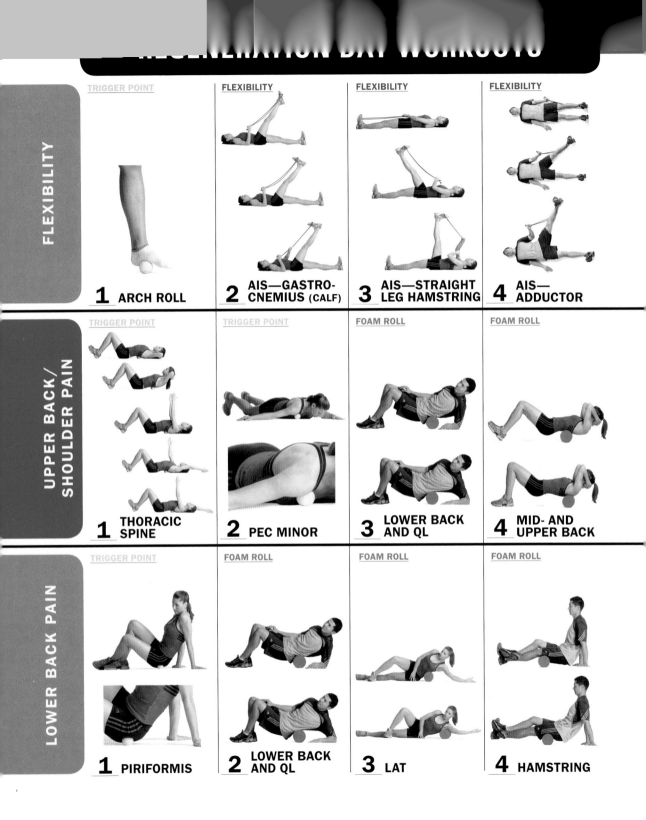

FLEXIBILITY

TRIGGER POINT
1 ARCH ROLL

FLEXIBILITY
2 AIS—GASTRO-CNEMIUS (CALF)

FLEXIBILITY
3 AIS—STRAIGHT LEG HAMSTRING

FLEXIBILITY
4 AIS—ADDUCTOR

UPPER BACK/SHOULDER PAIN

TRIGGER POINT
1 THORACIC SPINE

TRIGGER POINT
2 PEC MINOR

FOAM ROLL
3 LOWER BACK AND QL

FOAM ROLL
4 MID- AND UPPER BACK

LOWER BACK PAIN

TRIGGER POINT
1 PIRIFORMIS

FOAM ROLL
2 LOWER BACK AND QL

FOAM ROLL
3 LAT

FOAM ROLL
4 HAMSTRING

The routines below are for mild post-workout aches and pains. For persistent pain or acute injuries, consult a physician.

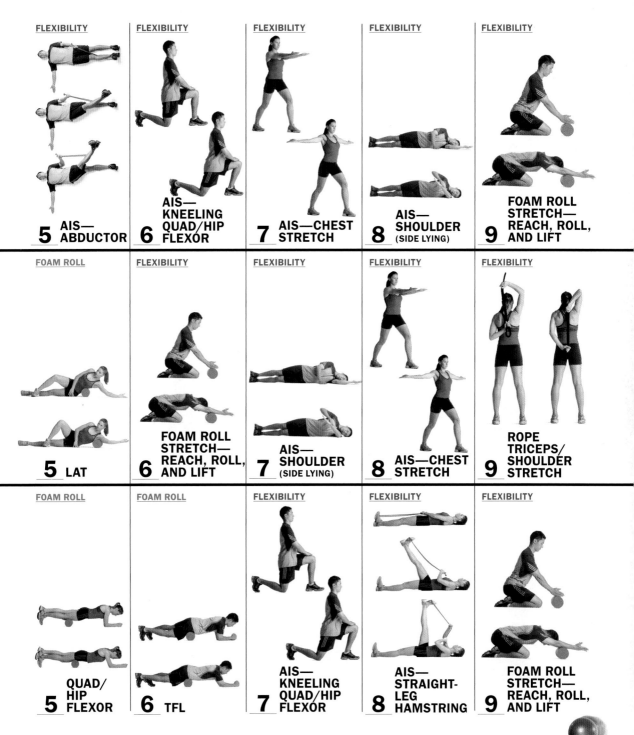

FLEXIBILITY

5 AIS— ABDUCTOR

FLEXIBILITY

6 AIS— KNEELING QUAD/HIP FLEXOR

FLEXIBILITY

7 AIS—CHEST STRETCH

FLEXIBILITY

8 AIS— SHOULDER (SIDE LYING)

FLEXIBILITY

9 FOAM ROLL STRETCH— REACH, ROLL, AND LIFT

FOAM ROLL

5 LAT

FLEXIBILITY

6 FOAM ROLL STRETCH— REACH, ROLL, AND LIFT

FLEXIBILITY

7 AIS— SHOULDER (SIDE LYING)

FLEXIBILITY

8 AIS—CHEST STRETCH

FLEXIBILITY

9 ROPE TRICEPS/ SHOULDER STRETCH

FOAM ROLL

5 QUAD/ HIP FLEXOR

FOAM ROLL

6 TFL

FLEXIBILITY

7 AIS— KNEELING QUAD/HIP FLEXOR

FLEXIBILITY

8 AIS— STRAIGHT- LEG HAMSTRING

FLEXIBILITY

9 FOAM ROLL STRETCH— REACH, ROLL, AND LIFT

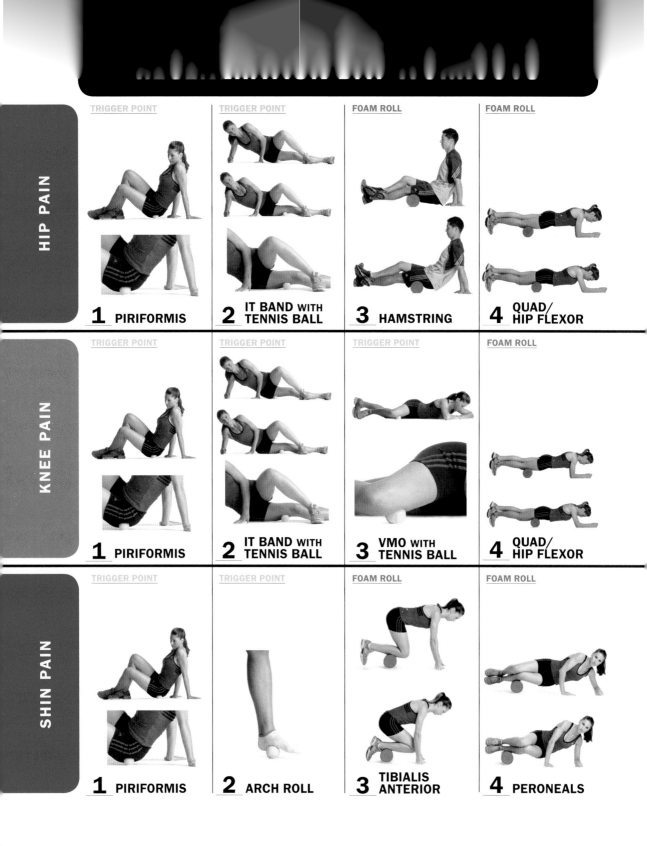

	TRIGGER POINT	TRIGGER POINT	FOAM ROLL	FOAM ROLL
HIP PAIN	**1** PIRIFORMIS	**2** IT BAND WITH TENNIS BALL	**3** HAMSTRING	**4** QUAD/ HIP FLEXOR
	TRIGGER POINT	TRIGGER POINT	TRIGGER POINT	FOAM ROLL
KNEE PAIN	**1** PIRIFORMIS	**2** IT BAND WITH TENNIS BALL	**3** VMO WITH TENNIS BALL	**4** QUAD/ HIP FLEXOR
	TRIGGER POINT	TRIGGER POINT	FOAM ROLL	FOAM ROLL
SHIN PAIN	**1** PIRIFORMIS	**2** ARCH ROLL	**3** TIBIALIS ANTERIOR	**4** PERONEALS

The routines below are for mild post-workout aches and pains. For persistent pain or acute injuries, consult a physician.

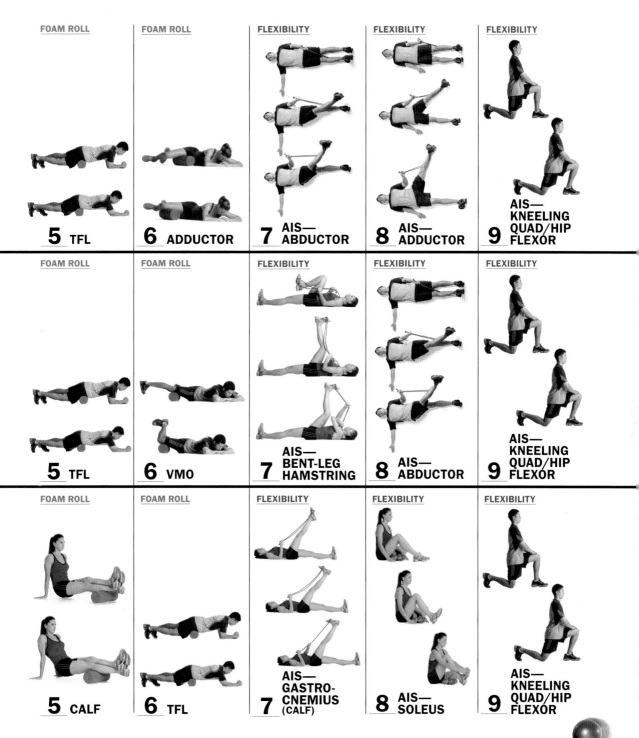

FOAM ROLL
5 TFL

FOAM ROLL
6 ADDUCTOR

FLEXIBILITY
7 AIS— ABDUCTOR

FLEXIBILITY
8 AIS— ADDUCTOR

FLEXIBILITY
9 AIS— KNEELING QUAD/HIP FLEXOR

FOAM ROLL
5 TFL

FOAM ROLL
6 VMO

FLEXIBILITY
7 AIS— BENT-LEG HAMSTRING

FLEXIBILITY
8 AIS— ABDUCTOR

FLEXIBILITY
9 AIS— KNEELING QUAD/HIP FLEXOR

FOAM ROLL
5 CALF

FOAM ROLL
6 TFL

FLEXIBILITY
7 AIS— GASTRO-CNEMIUS (CALF)

FLEXIBILITY
8 AIS— SOLEUS

FLEXIBILITY
9 AIS— KNEELING QUAD/HIP FLEXOR

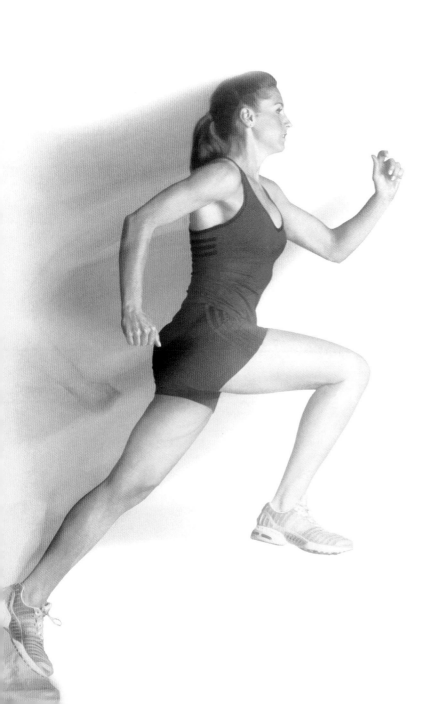

FAQs

Q: *I was told I should run on my toes to be fast. Is this correct?*

A: When most people think of running on their toes, they picture themselves keeping their heels off the ground. This is an old school myth—and an improper one. Running on your toes, or staying plantar flexed, will set you up for many common running ailments, including shinsplints, hamstring and hip flexor strains and tightness, and knee, hip, and lower back pain. It also will severely compromise your performance. Your body should remain in a vertical alignment, with your foot striking underneath your hip with a full foot landing, and a rollover on the ball of your foot through a pushoff over the big toe. This will allow you to decrease your injury potential and improve your performance.

Q: *I like to wake up and run on an empty stomach. Is this okay?*

A: No. If you wake up and run on an empty stomach, you are running in a completely fasted state, as your body has used up all of its energy in fueling your body for recovery overnight. When you wake up and go, your body does not have the proper fuel to power your run. Being resourceful, it will tap into your stored lean body mass first and your fat tissue second, which is counterproductive for staying healthy and performing at your best. Your body, in this stressed state, will release high amounts of the stress hormone cortisol, decreasing the overall benefit of your healthy adventure.

Instead of working out on an empty stomach, have a small, easily digestible mini-meal, even if it's just half a glass of water or watered-down orange juice with a scoop of whey protein. Other options include yogurt and water, an EAS Myoplex Lite ready-to-drink product, or a cup of coffee with some fat-free milk and a piece of whole wheat bread with jam. You'll be much better off in the, ahem, long run.

Q: *Is it normal to have knee pain for the first 15 minutes of my run before it goes away? I manage it with ice and ibuprofen after workouts.*

A: No, it's not normal. When your body hurts, it is trying to communicate with you, so listen. Let's provide the best long-term solution. Decrease your volume of running significantly and follow the Core Performance Endurance program to improve your mobility, stability, and running mechanics. Work the overall system for a few weeks, making sure to follow the regeneration strategies, and you'll decrease the pain. If the pain persists after a few weeks of this, seek out a respected sports physical therapist for some hands-on evaluation and treatment.

Q: *Why is posture important for swimmers?*

A: Just because your sport puts you in a horizontal position supported by the partial buoyancy of water, it's no excuse for poor posture. If you look at the form of most swimmers, you will see that the head is forward, the shoulders are rounded forward, the thumbs point in toward the middle of the body, and the back is S-shaped. Over time, this position will cause shoulder problems. Why? Because your body adapts to the high-volume, repetitive work in these similar movements that cause internal rotation, creating muscle imbalances.

By focusing on your posture and developing pillar strength, you will decrease your potential for injury, as well as improving your performance, because you will better link your upper and lower body. This is the secret of world-class swimmers: Their shoulders and hips counter-rotate, which stores energy throughout their pillar, and they utilize this for subsequent strokes that are faster and more efficient. Develop your pillar strength, and you'll be amazed at the results.

Q: *Won't strength training make me big?*

A: The goal of the Core Performance system is not to develop useless big muscles. Our goal is more akin to tuning a high-performance car. We follow movement patterns and strength programs designed to develop speed, power, and strength, not size. Our goal is to tune you like that high-performance car, shaving unnecessary weight in the form of body fat and unused muscles, and increase your pound-for-pound speed, power, and endurance. Stick with this program, and you will notice improved performance with minimal increase in muscle size, but increased muscle function and tone.

Q: *I'm not hungry after my workout, but I know I should eat. What's the easiest solution?*

A: Follow that instinct to eat. Immediately after your workout, your muscle cells are screaming for nutrients and energy to replace those lost through exercise. You want to refill your tank immediately, ideally within 10 minutes after your workout. Find something that is convenient—preferably a liquid, to assist in hydration and digest rapidly so that your muscles get what they want. Examples of this may be a post-workout supplement such as EAS Endurathon, Gatorade Pro, or Amino Vital. Then, within the next 30 to 60 minutes, grab a meal consisting of your favorite nutritious foods. (See the list in Part 3 of this book.)

Q: *Will this program help with common running ailments or help to correct bad form?*

A: Yes. Everything in this program is geared toward building proper stability and pillar strength. The program retrains your body to move more efficiently and effectively. You'll regain the flexibility and mobility you had as a child. All of these things will produce more fluid, proper movement that will correct bad form and prevent common running ailments.

Q: *Is static stretching really bad?*

A: Static stretching can be a great tool, when properly timed. The Core Performance philosophy stresses that the warmup, what we call Movement Prep, is active and dynamic. This does not make static stretching bad. Static stretching works by sending a message to the muscle saying, "Shut this tightness off," and it ultimately forces the muscle to release through these static stretches, which are akin to submissive wrestling holds. Static stretching is best used post-workout or later on that day or night to elongate the muscle and connective tissue, while turning off the overachieving nervous system. It is also effective on pure recovery days, even before you do a warmup. Long static holds help to produce long-term changes in the fascia (the band of elastic tissue that envelops the body, beneath the skin), ultimately improving muscle balance and length.

Q: *When should I take time off?*

A: Proactively, as part of your plan. The endurance culture is to keep going and going, but ultimately, your body will revolt in the form of a slight strain or even a major injury because you have been ignoring all of its signals. It's best to schedule time off into each week, month, and year as prescribed in this book. When you adopt this type of planning, you will continue to improve systematically, avoiding injuries, and you will watch your performance improve. It's your choice—proactively or reactively; but either way, you will have to take the time off. Why not do it on your terms?

Q: *How much is too much?*

A: Most endurance athletes think that more training is better. But that's not really true. *Better* training is better. If you are not sleeping well at night, don't have much energy, suffer from chronic illness because your immune system is depressed, have stiff or achy muscles and joints, or are generally grumpy, *you are doing too much.* Most programs focus on very high volume. Try cutting your volume in half and see whether your

performance improves or declines. Chances are, it will improve.

Q: *What do I do if something starts to hurt?*

A: Immediately start to identify what exactly is hurting, then apply many of the concepts we discuss in the book. Examine your biomechanics, your symmetry from right to left, your pillar strength—and the inner workings of all the systems we discuss. Stop doing what hurts, and embark on 3 to 7 days of a regeneration-focused training plan. If the pain has subsided for some time, gradually start training with low volume and take regenerative days off between activity.

If the pain persists, seek out a qualified sports physical therapist for a hands-on evaluation and treatment. It's much easier to deal with the small stuff than to turn a blind eye and set yourself up for a major injury.

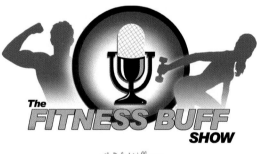

AFTERWORD

I n my previous books, *Core Performance* and *Core Performance Essentials,* I issued a challenge to readers to send us their feedback about the program. I've heard from many wonderful people who have used the Core system to overcome pain, lose weight, increase flexibility, and install a plan of high-performance nutrition and exercise for long-term health and success.

I'm especially excited to hear from readers of this book. One of the greatest rewards in my career has been to take highly motivated people and show them how to become even better. I'm guessing that when you picked up this book, you already had achieved some incredible endurance feats. Maybe you've completed marathons or triathlons. Perhaps you've excelled at cycling or swimming. With this program, I'm confident you'll raise the level of your performance even higher. You'll do so pain-free, with a system in place that will ensure not only your excellence in endurance sports but also your long-term health.

This system will last you the rest of your endurance career, which can be the rest of your life. No longer must you accept a decline in performance as a result of age. With this system, there's no reason you can't get better as you get older. That's why the progressions in the Core Performance Endurance system are endless. Life is an ongoing process. You'll notice that we did not put a timeframe on this program. There's no "12 Weeks to a Better You" slogan, no "6-Week Plan for Success" subtitle. This program has infinite progressions.

This book might be all you ever need to complement your endurance training, but I'd like to give you some other low-cost options that will enhance your performance exponentially.

Thousands of people have joined our online community at www.coreperformance.com/endurance. Each week, we answer questions about the Core program and provide them with the latest scientific information on nutrition, fitness, and performance. I hope you'll join this growing community of people who have made the commitment to a lifetime of high performance.

We assembled this program with the goal of using as little equipment as possible, recognizing that endurance athletes often have only a modest amount of space in their training bag or bike box. We wanted to eliminate excuses for not following this system, while providing an efficient program that will allow you to succeed regardless of your financial resources. By following this program, you will achieve great results.

But since we've saved you the cost of a monthly gym membership, perhaps you have a little more money to spend. And, if you do, there are some tools we provide that can help you train even more efficiently and reach your endurance goals.

This book's Web site is the home for the products and programs we have developed and tested that will complement your Core training program. Go to www.coreperformance.com/endurance.

First, check out our online Core Store. We have assembled several tools, based on the book, that are great resources for the Core Performance Endurance program, whether you prefer to work out at home or in a gym. I know many of you have told me that you love our workouts, and I wish I could be there to lead you through them. Well, along those lines, we have created a Core Performance DVD series, in which I lead you through the various 30-minute workouts right in your living room.

Alternatively, you'll find in the Core Store a set of laminated cards featuring each level of the workouts with exercise pictures. These cards are a great tool to remind you of proper form as you work out at home or the gym.

Also in the Core Store, we have assembled several packages to create a Core Gym at home. I know that you are incredibly busy, and maybe a gym membership is just not feasible, or maybe you have a membership but are never able to use it for lack of time.

Maybe you prefer to train wherever you run, swim, or cycle. A simple Core home gym lets you build the Core program around *your* life.

Maybe you're thinking, "Sure, that would be great, but I don't have the time or space for elaborate equipment." The beauty of this is that the equipment is easy to use and compact. It will fit under your bed or in a small corner of a room.

Our equipment partner, GoFit, has teamed with us to compile several affordable packages of equipment that you can purchase in the Core Store. Of course, you also can purchase individual pieces of equipment to fit your needs.

Once you've checked out the Core Store, you will notice a whole world of Core Performance programs available on the Web site. If you're new to the Core Performance community and just beginning to take charge of your body and your life, I want you to focus on this book and mastering the program. We tried to make this book all-encompassing, and indeed, if you just keep trying to pack more and more into your Core workouts, this book might be all you ever need.

But if you're like most endurance athletes I know, you're probably someone who wants to take your game to higher levels. If you're one of these people, check out the programs on the Web site.

The Core Store also offers the original *Core Performance* book (now in paperback), and the sequel *Core Performance Essentials,* which was designed for the time-pressed person competing in the Game of Life. The Core Store also offers sport-specific DVD training systems for golf, soccer, tennis, football, and baseball. Each of these DVDs contains a program with more than 60 exercises designed to help you prepare to thrive in each of these sports. These are great products if you're a competitive or recreational athlete, and I have even recommended them with great success to professional athletes who cannot join us at our Athletes' Performance Institutes.

I also recommend that you check out our powerful interactive platform, which can be accessed from www.coreperformance.com/endurance. We created this platform based on feedback from readers of the original *Core Performance* who were looking for more progressions to the workout. This interactive platform features Core Performance programs for different levels of fitness and 15 sports. My staff and I assembled these programs in a powerful database, all customized to your goals, interests, and life's demands based on simple questions that you answer.

There is a complete nutritional system that complements your customized training program, providing you with recommendations on meal timing and food choices as part of your customized "Perfect Day" routine. We have effective visual tools that let you track and monitor your progress. There are video clips of every exercise. And I try to provide you with daily tips and world-class content that reflect the constantly evolving research and development we do at the Athletes' Performance Institutes every day.

In short, www.coreperformance.com/endurance is the next best thing to being here in person.

I also encourage you to visit the Web site of another one of my partners, Active.com, which is the best online resource to learn about and register for endurance competitions. Active.com provides information on an endless number of events for you to showcase your new Core Performance strategies.

Ultimately, I want you to be members of the Core Performance online community for life, which is why we have made a full-year membership available for less than the cost of a weekly cup of coffee. This means that for the cost of a personal training session, you will have progressive programs that are based upon your lifestyles and accomplishments and that can change with you as your goals and demands change.

Even better, because you have made a commitment to joining the Core community, I am providing you with a free 3-week trial to try out the site. From www.coreperformance.com/endurance, simply click on "Enter Your Code" and type in the following code: CPE20495. You'll have 3 weeks to sample the programs, check out all of the amazing tools on the site, and decide whether you want to become a member.

I've had great success supporting people in the pursuit of their dreams. Some of them are prominent sports figures, but many of them are people just like you who have reached spectacular goals. What I love most is being able to build my athletes, to see them evolve and reach their goals.

I'm excited about this book because I will get to hear from more people like you, and that inspires me. Many of you have become vocal advocates for this program, and I can't tell you how much I appreciate that.

I want to hear how this program has transformed your endurance training—and not just from a physical standpoint. Tell me how it has enabled you to meet challenges, overcome injuries, and fulfill your dreams. I want to hear about what you've overcome and the roadblocks you've navigated. Tell the entire Core community how taking a proactive approach to life has made a difference.

Please share your stories with us at mark@coreperformance.com. We'll pick the most inspirational submissions, the ones that touch us the most, and bring the authors of those remarks to one of the Athletes'

Performance Institutes to train in person with our staff, alongside some of the best athletes in the world.

Let's help each other stay motivated through the Web site, where you can progress based upon your goals. You will empower me through your achievements and courage. You can share with me personally how you've transformed your life to meet your goals, motivating me even further.

We can't bring everyone out, unfortunately. I hope you join our online community and interact with the growing number of people dedicated to treating each day as an athletic event and properly preparing themselves for the competition that is the Game of Life.

Welcome to the enduring world of Core Performance.

Your coach,

Mark Verstegen

ACKNOWLEDGMENTS

Writing a book is an endurance sport, and I could not have finished the race without help from a talented team of people.

As always, the staff, athletes, and extended family of the Athletes' Performance Institutes have both inspired this project and made significant contributions. A very special thanks goes to Amanda Carlson, Craig Friedman, Darcy Norman, Paul Robbins, Dan Burns, and Scott Peltin for helping to shape the message of this endurance program. I also owe a huge debt of gratitude to my co-conspirators Pete Williams and David Black, along with Rodale's ever-supportive team of Zach Schisgal, Pete Fornatale, Kathy LeSage, Susan Eugster, Karen Neely, and Susannah Hogendorn. As for my wife, Amy, no words can express my gratitude for your enduring support.

INDEX

Boldface page references indicate photographs.
<u>Underscored</u> references indicate boxed text.

A

Abdominal muscles, 29, 30
Abductor, AIS, 187, **187**
Active-isolated stretching (AIS)
    exercises
  abductor, 187, **187**
  adductor, 188, **188**
  bent-leg hamstring, 184, **184**
  chest stretch, 189, **189**
  gastrocnemius (calf), 182, **182**
  kneeling quad/hip flexor, 186,
    186
  rope use with, 55–57
  shoulder (side lying), 190, **190**
  soleus, 183, **183**
  straight-leg hamstring, 185,
    185
Adductor
  AIS (active-isolated stretching),
    188, **188**
  foam roll exercise, 177, **177**

Aerobic base, <u>46</u>
Aerobic zone, 44–45, 48
AIS. *See* Active-isolated stretching
    (AIS) exercises
Alactate power, 43, 44
Alcohol, 81, 82
Amenorrhea, <u>63</u>
Amino acids
  branched chain (BCAAs),
    96–97
  glutamine, 97–98, **98–99**
  leucine, **98–99**
Amino Vital Endurance, 80–82,
    86, <u>94</u>, 95, 217
Anaerobic energy system, 43,
    44
Antioxidants, 66, 81, 95, **96–97**,
    97
Apple, 90, 93
Arch roll, 193, **193**
Arm action, in running, 18–21, **19**

B

Back
  foam roll exercise, for
    lower back, 179, **179**
    mid- and upper back, 180,
      180
  pain, regeneration workout for,
    210–11
Bagel, 90, 93
Banana, 90, 93, 95
BCAAs, **96–97**
Bench press
  dumbbell, 170, **170**
  dumbbell, alternating, 163, **163**
Bent-over *Y*s and *L*s, 146–47,
    146–47
Bike fit, <u>33</u>
Blood flow
  in capillaries, 44, 48
  stimulation with hot and cold
    contrasts, 57

Blood glucose
glycemic index, <u>67</u>, <u>68–69</u>
race day levels, 92
Bone density, 62
Box hop, linear, 149, **149**
Branched chain amino acids
(BCAAs), **96–97**
Breakfast, 77

C

Cable crossover, standing, 145,
145
Cable row
one-leg squat to, 167, **167**
Romanian deadlift to, 161, **161**
Cadence, running, <u>36</u>
Caffeine, 81, 82, **96–97**, 99–100
Calcium, 70, **96–97**
Calendar, Core Performance, 199
Calf
AIS (active-isolated stretching),
182, **182**
foam roll exercise, 171, **171**
Capillaries, 44, 48
Carbohydrate-electrolyte drinks,
81, 82, 86, 93
Carbohydrate loading, <u>91</u>
Carbohydrates
consumption
event day, 92–93, 95
post-event/post-training, 89,
95
training day, 86–87
as fuels, 65–66
glycemic index, 66, <u>67</u>, <u>68–69</u>
low-carb diet, 65, 66, <u>66</u>
in meal-replacement bars, <u>76</u>
performance points, 68
processed, 66
quantity, 66, 68
sources of, 89–91, 93
supplements, **96–97**
types, 66
Cardio, 43, <u>46–47</u>. See also
Energy System
Development (ESD)

Casein, **98–99**
Catabolic state, 64, 70
Catapult, 100
Cereals, 90, 93
Chest stretch, AIS, 189, **189**
Chicken, 70, <u>78</u>
Cholesterol
LDL and HDL, 71
lowering with nuts, 74
raising with saturated fats, 71
Clif Bar, 91
Clif Shot, 86, 91, 95
Cod, 70
Cold therapy, 57
Compression, deep, 54–55
Contrasts, 57
Core stability, 29–30
Corn syrup, high-fructose, <u>76</u>, 81
Cortisol, 87, 215
Cottage cheese, 71
Craving, food, <u>52</u>
Cycling
bike fit, <u>33</u>
dorsiflexion in, 15
force transfer, 20
glute strength for hip stability,
29
revolutions per minute (RPMs),
<u>36</u>
Cytomax, 80, 86, 91, 95

D

Dairy products
low-fat, 70
whole-fat, 71
Dehydration, 80
Diabetes, reduced risk with low-
glycemic diets, <u>68</u>, <u>69</u>
Diet, low-carb, 65, 66, <u>66</u>
Dorsiflexion, 13–17
Drinks
shakes, post-workout recovery,
70, 71, 86–87, 95
shooter, pre-workout, 86, 87
sports, 80, 81–82, 95
Drop squat and stabilize, 150, **150**

E

EAS
Catapult, 100
Endurathon, 80, 81, 86, 217
Myoplex products, 86, 91, 95,
98, 216
Eating. See Nutrition
Eggs, 71
Elasticity
energy storage and release, 3,
36, 37
exercises (see Exercises,
elasticity)
stability and mobility as
foundation of, 3–4
tissue tolerance, 4–6
workouts
power day, level 1, 200,
200–201
power day, level 2, 202,
202–3
Electrolytes
carbohydrate-electrolyte drinks,
81, 82, 86, 93
loss in water intoxication, <u>94</u>
Endurathon (EAS), 80, 81, 86,
217
Energy
aerobic system, 43–45, 48–49
anaerobic system, 43, 44
leaks, 37
recycling, 36, 37
Energy System Development
(ESD)
aerobic energy system, 43–45,
48–49
anaerobic energy system, 43,
44
power days, 109–10, 200, 202
regeneration days, 114, 209
strength days, 110, 112–13,
204, 206
Exercises
elasticity
double-contact hurdle hop,
154–55, **154–55**

drop squat and stabilize, 150, **150**

lateral bound—quick/ stabilize, 152–53, **152–53**

linear box hop, 149, **149**

mini band lateral bound— stabilization, 148, **148**

reactive stepup, 157, **157**

squat jump— countermovement, 156, **156**

squat jump—non- countermovement, 151, **151**

movement prep

backward lunge with lateral flexion (in place), 123, **123**

backward lunge with lateral flexion (moving), 130–31, **130–31**

drop lunge, 132–33, **132–33**

forward lunge, elbow to instep (crawling), 120, **120**

forward lunge, elbow to instep (walking), 127, **127**

inverted hamstring stretch, 119, **119**

inverted hamstring stretch (backward), 126, **126**

knee hug (in place), 121, **121**

knee hug (moving), 128, **128**

leg cradle, 124, **124**

pillar march (moving), 122, **122**

pillar skip (in place), 129, **129**

quadruped posterior rocking, 125, **125**

reverse 90/90 stretch, 118, **118**

prehab

bent-over Ys and Ls, 146–47, **146–47**

floor Ys, 140, **140**

four-way hip cable, 138–39, **138–39**

front pillar with diagonal arm lift, 141, **141**

glute bridge marching (hip flexion), 143, **143**

glute bridge marching (knee extension), 136, **136**

lateral pillar (abduction), 142, **142**

mini band bent-knee walk, 144, **144**

mini band internal/external rotation, 137, **137**

pillar bridge front, 134, **134**

pillar bridge lateral—feet split, 135, **135**

standing cable crossover, 145, **145**

regeneration, flexibility exercises

AIS abductor, 187, **187**

AIS adductor, 188, **188**

AIS bent-leg hamstring, 184, **184**

AIS chest stretch, 189, **189**

AIS gastrocnemius (calf), 182, **182**

AIS kneeling quad/hip flexor, 186, **186**

AIS shoulder (side lying), 190, **190**

AIS soleus, 183, **183**

AIS straight-leg hamstring, 185, **185**

foam roll stretch—reach, roll, and lift, 192, **192**

rope triceps/shoulder stretch, 191, **191**

regeneration, foam roll exercises

adductor, 177, **177**

calf, 171, **171**

hamstring, 174, **174**

lat (latissimus dorsi), 181, **181**

lower back and QL (quadratus lumborum), 179, **179**

mid- and upper back, 180, **180**

peroneals, 172, **172**

quad/hip flexor, 175, **175**

TFL (tensor fasciae latae), 178, **178**

tibialis anterior, 173, **173**

VMO (vastus medialis obliquus), 176, **176**

regeneration, trigger point exercises

arch roll, 193, **193**

IT (iliotibial) band with tennis ball, 195, **195**

pec minor, 194, **194**

piriformis, 196, **196**

thoracic spine, 198, **198**

VMO (vastus medialis obliquus) with tennis ball, 197, **197**

strength

dumbbell bench press, 170, **170**

dumbbell bench press— alternating, 163, **163**

half-kneeling high cable stability chop, 158, **158**

half-kneeling low cable stability lift, 159, **159**

high cable split stability chop, 164, **164**

low cable split stability lift, 165, **165**

one-leg squat to cable row, 167, **167**

Romanian deadlift to cable row, 161, **161**

Valslide eccentric leg curl, 160, **160**

Valslide lateral squat, 168, **168**

Valslide leg curl, 166, **166**

Exercises (*cont.*)
    Valslide or regular split
        squat, 162, **162**
    Valslide pushup, 169, **169**

F

Fat, dietary
  performance points, 74–75
  race day consumption of, 93
  roles of, 71
  saturated, 71
  trans, 71, 74
  unsaturated, 74
Fatty acids, essential, **98–99**
Female athlete triad, 63
Fiber, 66, 69, 76, 93
Fish, 70, 74, 77
Fish oil, 74, 95
Flaxseed oil, 74
Flexibility
  exercises
    AIS abductor, 187, **187**
    AIS adductor, 188, **188**
    AIS bent-leg hamstring, 184,
      184
    AIS chest stretch, 189, **189**
    AIS gastrocnemius (calf),
      182, **182**
    AIS kneeling quad/hip flexor,
      186, **186**
    AIS shoulder (side lying),
      190, **190**
    AIS soleus, 183, **183**
    AIS straight-leg hamstring,
      185, **185**
    foam roll stretch—reach,
      roll, and lift, 192, **192**
    rope triceps/shoulder
      stretch, 191, **191**
  regeneration workout for,
    210–11
Flushing, 44, 114
Foam roll exercises
  adductor, 177, **177**
  calf, 171, **171**
  hamstring, 174, **174**

lat (latissimus dorsi), 181, **181**
lower back and QL (quadratus
    lumborum), 179, **179**
as massage, 54–55
mid- and upper back, 180, **180**
peroneals, 172, **172**
quad/hip flexor, 175, **175**
TFL (tensor fasciae latae), 178,
    178
tibialis anterior, 173, **173**
VMO (vastus medialis
    obliquus), 176, **176**
Food. *See also* Nutrition
  glycemic index, 66, 67, 68–69
  grocery list, 72–73
  serving sizes, 73
Four-way hip cable, 138–39,
    138–39
Free radical, 66
Front pillar with diagonal arm lift,
    141, **141**
Fruits, 90, 93

G

Gastrocnemius, AIS, 182, **182**
Gatorade, 80–82, 86, 91, 93, 94,
    95, 217
GatorLytes, 94
Glucose
  content of sports drinks, 80
  glycemic index, 67, 68–69
Glutamine, 97–98, **98–99**
Glute bridge
  marching (hip flexion), 143,
    143
  marching (knee extension),
    136, **136**
Glutes, strong for hip stability,
    28–29
Glycemic index, 66, 67, 68–69
Glycogen, 94, 99
Go-Fit Pro Gym-in-a-Bag, 111
Grains, 90, 93
Grocery list, 72–73
Growth hormone, 53
Gu, 86, 93, 94, 95

H

Hammer Gel, 86, 94, 95
Hamstrings
  bent-leg AIS (active-isolated
    stretching), 184,
    184
  foam roll exercise, 174, **174**
  straight-leg AIS (active-isolated
    stretching), 185, **185**
  stretch, inverted, 119, **119**
  stretch, inverted (backward),
    126, **126**
  tightness, 16, 215
HDL cholesterol, 71
Heart disease
  increased risk with saturated
    fats, 71
  reduced risk with
    low-glycemic diets, 68, 69
    nuts, 74
Heart rate
  monitor, 46
  training zones, 46–47, 49
Heel strike, shinsplints and, 20
Hip
  pain, regeneration workout for,
    212–13
  stability, 28–29
Hip cable, four-way, 138–39,
    138–39
Hip flexor
  foam roll exercise, 175,
    175
  kneeling AIS, 186, **186**
Hot and cold contrasts, 57
Hurdle hop, double-contact,
    154–55, **154–55**
Hydration
  performance points, 82
  race day, 92, 94–95
  sports drinks, 80, 81–82,
    95
  training day, 85, 87
  water, 80
Hydrogen ions, 37, 45
Hyponatremia, 94

I

Imbalances, 12, 28, 216
Inflammation, decrease with cold therapy, 57
Interval training, 46–47
IT (iliotibial) band, trigger point exercise, 195, **195**

J

Juice, 82, 90–91, 93

K

Kinetic chain, 40
Knee hug
  moving, 128, **128**
  in place, 121, **121**
Knee pain
  regeneration workout for, **212–13**
  while running, 216
Knots, tissue, 55

L

Lactate, 37, 45, 48
Lactate threshold, 43–45, 48–49
Lat (latissimus dorsi), foam roll exercise, 181, **181**
Lateral bound—quick/stabilize, 152–53, **152–53**
Lateral pillar (abduction), 142, **142**
LDL cholesterol, 71
Leg cradle, 124, **124**
Leg curl
  Valslide, 166, **166**
  Valslide eccentric, 160, **160**
Leucine, **98–99**
Lower back
  foam roll exercise, 179, **179**
  pain, regeneration workout for, **210–11**
Lunge
  backward with lateral flexion (in place), 123, **123**
  backward with lateral flexion (moving), 130–31, **130–31**

drop, 132–33, **132–33**
forward, elbow to instep (crawling), 120, **120**
forward, elbow to instep (walking), 127, **127**

M

Massage
  foam roll routine as, 54–55
  self-massage regeneration workout, **208–9**
Meal-replacement bars, 76
Meals
  3-for-3 formula, 75, 77, 80
  assembly, 78–79
  balanced, 77
  number and frequency, 75, 77
  plans for male and female athletes, 78
  pre-event, 89
Meat, lean red, 70, 71
Menstrual period, 63
Metabolism, boost with
  frequent meals, 75
  protein consumption, 70
Milk, 71, 91, 216
Mini band exercises
  bent-knee walk, 144, **144**
  internal/external rotation, 137, **137**
  lateral bound—stabilization, 148, **148**
Mitochondria, 44, 48
Mobility, 4
Movement dysfunctions, 5
Movement preparation
  benefits of, 26–27
  exercises (*See* Exercises, movement prep)
  workouts
    power day, level 1, 200, **200–201**
    power day, level 2, 202, **202–3**

strength day, level 1, 204, **204–5**
strength day, level 2, 206, **206–7**
Multivitamin, 95, **98–99**
Muscle(s)
  glycogen, 94, 99
  loss, 75
  microtears in, 57
  recruitment of, 35–36, 40
  spasms, 55
  stabilizer, 29, 39
Myoplex products, 86, 91, 95, 98

N

National Sleep Foundation, 52
Nutrition
  for balanced body, 64, 65, 75
  carbohydrates, 65–68
  event day
    categories, 87
    during competition, 94–95
    planning, 92
    post-event, 89–91, 95
    pre-event food choices, 92–93
    pre-event sample meals, 89
    timing, 88
  fat, 71, 74–75
  female athlete triad, 63
  grocery list, 72–73
  hydration, 80–82
  importance to endurance athletes, 61–62, 64–65
  meal frequency, 75, 77
  protein, 69–71
  running on empty stomach, 215–16
  supplements, 95–100, **96–99**
  training day
    after workout, 64, 86–87, 89–91, 217
    before workout, 86
    during workout, 86
    performance points, 87
Nuts, 74

O

Oatmeal, 74
Oils, blended, 74
Olive oil, 77
Omega-3 fatty acid, 70, 74
Omega-6 fatty acid, 70, 74
Osteoporosis, 63
Oxygen
  aerobic energy system, 43–45,
    48–49
  VO_2, max, 45, 46, 48

P

Pain
  dealing with, 218
  regeneration workouts for
    hip, **212–13**
    knee, **212–13**
    lower back, **210–11**
    shin, **212–13**
    upper back/shoulder,
      210–11
  while running, 216
Pasta, 77
Pec minor, trigger point exercise,
  194, **194**
Performance, hydration for, 80
Peroneals, foam roll exercise for,
  172, **172**
Pillar bridge
  front, 134, **134**
  lateral—feet split, 135, **135**
Pillar march (moving), 122, **122**
Pillar skip (in place), 129, **129**
Pillar strength
  as foundation of movement,
    27
  for power production, 37
  for swimmers, 216
Piriformis, trigger point exercise
  for, 196, **196**
Pork, 70
Posture
  running, 32
  shoulder, 30–31, **31**
  swimming, 216

Power
  alactate, 43, 44
  elasticity as component of, 36
  importance for endurance
    athletes, 35–37
  workouts
    description of workout,
      109–10
    heart rate training zone for,
      47
    level 1, 200, **200–201**
    level 2, 202, **202–3**
PowerBar, 91, 93
Prehabilitation
  benefits, 31–33
  exercises (See Exercises,
    prehab)
  pillar strength development,
    27–28
  workouts
    power day, level 1, 200,
      200–201
    power day, level 2, 202,
      202–3
Proprioception, improved with
  movement preparation, 26
Propulsion, strength for, 40–41
Protein
  meal-replacement bars, 76
  performance points, 71
  requirements, 69–70, 71
  roles of, 69
  shakes, 70, 71
  sources of, 70–71
  training day consumption,
    86–87
Pushup, Valslide, 169, **169**

Q

QL (quadratus lumborum), foam
  roll exercise for, 179, **179**
Quad/hip flexor
  foam roll exercise, 175, **175**
  kneeling AIS, 186, **186**
Quadruped posterior rocking,
  125, **125**

R

Raisins, 90, 93
Recovery, 51. *See also*
    Regeneration
Regeneration
  active, 54
  benefits of, 54
  Energy System Development
    (ESD), 114, 209
  flexibility exercises
    AIS abductor, 187, **187**
    AIS adductor, 188, **188**
    AIS bent-leg hamstring, 184,
      184
    AIS chest stretch, 189, **189**
    AIS gastrocnemius (calf),
      182, **182**
    AIS kneeling quad/hip flexor,
      186, **186**
    AIS shoulder (side lying),
      190, **190**
    AIS soleus, 183, **183**
    AIS straight-leg hamstring,
      185, **185**
    foam roll stretch—reach,
      roll, and lift, 192, **192**
    rope triceps/shoulder
      stretch, 191, **191**
  foam roll exercises
    adductor, 177, **177**
    calf, 171, **171**
    hamstring, 174, **174**
    lat (latissimus dorsi), 181,
      181
    lower back and QL
      (quadratus lumborum),
      179, **179**
    as massage, 54–55
    mid- and upper back, 180, **180**
    peroneals, 172, **172**
    quad/hip flexor, 175, **175**
    TFL (tensor fasciae latae),
      178, **178**
    tibialis anterior, 173, **173**
    VMO (vastus medialis
      obliquus), 176, **176**

importance to success, 51–57
passive, 54
trigger point exercises
 arch roll, 193, **193**
 IT (iliotibial) band with tennis
  ball, 195, **195**
 pec minor, 194, **194**
 piriformis, 196, **196**
 thoracic spine, 198, **198**
 VMO (vastus medialis
  obliquus) with tennis ball,
  197, **197**
workouts
 aerobic zone, 45
 heart rate training zone, 46
Reverse 90/90 stretch, 118, **118**
Rice, brown, 77
Romanian deadlift to cable row,
 161, **161**
Rope, for AIS exercises, 55–57
Rope triceps/shoulder stretch,
 191, **191**
Running
 cadence, 36
 dorsiflexion in, 13–15
 on empty stomach, 215–16
 glute strength for hip stability,
  28–29
 posture, 32
 on toes, 215

S

Salmon, 70, 77
Seeds, 74
Self-evaluation
 arm action, 18–21, **19**
 bridges, **16–17**, 16–18
  straight-leg bridge,
   dorsiflexed, **16**
  straight-leg bridge, marching,
   dorsiflexed, **17**
  straight-leg bridge, marching,
   plantar-flexed, **17**
  straight-leg bridge, plantar-
   flexed, **16**
 dorsiflexion, 13–17

triple flexion response, 11–14,
 13–15
Serving sizes, 73
Shakes, post-workout recovery,
 70, 71, 86–87, 95
Shin pain
 regeneration workout for,
  212–13
 types of shinsplints, 20
Shooter, pre-workout, 86, 87
Shoulder
 AIS (side lying), 190, **190**
 pain, regeneration workout for,
  210–11
 shrug, 31
 stability, 30–31
Sleep
 deprivation, 52, 53
 number, 56
 stages, 52–53
Slideboard, 111. *See also*
  Valslide
Snacks
 between-meal, 76
 race-day, 93–94
Soda, 81, 82
Sodium
 hyponatremia, 94
 in sports drinks, 80, 81
Soleus, AIS, 183, **183**
Speed, loss with dehydration, 80
Sports drinks, 80, 81–82, 95
Squat
 drop squat and stabilize, 150,
  150
 one-leg squat to cable row,
  167, **167**
 Valslide lateral, 168, **168**
 Valslide or regular split, 162,
  162
Squat jump
 countermovement, 156, **156**
 non-countermovement, 151, **151**
Stability
 core, 29–30
 elasticity and, 3–4

hip, 28–29
rotary, 38
shoulder, 30–31
strength for, 39–40
Stability chop
 half-kneeling high cable, 158,
  158
 high cable split, 164, **164**
Stability lift
 half-kneeling low cable, 159, **159**
 low cable split, 165, **165**
Stabilizer muscles, 29, 39
Stage training system, 46–47
Starches, 90
Stepup, reactive, 157, **157**
Strength
 circuit workouts
  strength day, level 1, 204,
   204–5
  strength day, level 2, 206,
   206–7
 exercises (*See* Exercises,
  strength)
 loss with dehydration, 80
 muscle size and, 216–17
 types
  functional, 38
  propulsive, 40–41
  relative, 38
  stabilizing, 39–40
Stretching. *See also* Movement
  preparation
 AIS (*See* Active-isolated
  stretching (AIS) exercises)
 foam roll stretch—reach, roll,
  and lift, 192, **192**
 inverted hamstring stretch,
  119, **119**
 inverted hamstring stretch
  (backward), 126, **126**
 post-workout, 217
 prerace, 25–26
 reverse 90/90, 118, **118**
 rope triceps/shoulder stretch,
  191, **191**
 static, 25–26, 217

Stride, strike zone of, 16
Supplements, 95–100, **96–99**
Sweat
    sodium loss in, 80, 81
    water loss in, 94–95
Sweets, 91
Swimming
    body movement, 20–21
    efficiency, 39
    posture, importance of, 216
Swolf (swimming golf), 39
Symmetry, 12, 26

T
Tea, 80, 81
Testosterone, 87
TFL (tensor fasciae latae), foam
        roll exercise, 178, **178**
Thoracic spine, trigger point
        exercise for, 198, **198**
Tibialis anterior, foam roll
        exercise, 173, **173**
Tissue
    quality, 55
    spasms and knots, 55
    tolerance, 4–6
Tofu, 71
Training. See also Workouts
    interval, 46–47
    time off from, 217
Training zones, heart rate, 46–47,
        49
Transverse abdominis, 30
Trigger point exercises
    arch roll, 193, **193**
    IT (iliotibial) band with tennis
        ball, 195, **195**
    pec minor, 194, **194**
    piriformis, 196, **196**

thoracic spine, 198, **198**
VMO (vastus medialis obliquus)
        with tennis ball, 197, **197**
Triple flexion response, 11–14,
        13–15, 18, 20
Tuna, 70

U
Udo's Choice Blend, 74
University of Chicago Medical
        Center, 52
Upper back pain, regeneration
        workout for, **210–11**

V
Valslide
    exercises
        eccentric leg curl, 160, **160**
        lateral squat, 168, **168**
        leg curl, 166, **166**
        pushup, 169, **169**
        split squat, 162, **162**
    substitutes for, 111
Vegetables
    carbohydrates in, 90
    colorful, 77
    starchy, 90
Vitamins, 70, 95, 96, **96–99**
VMO (vastus medialis obliquus)
    foam roll exercise, 176, **176**
    trigger point exercise, 197,
        197
VO$_2$
    analyzer, 46, 49, **49**
    max, 45, 46, 48

W
Water intoxication, 94
Wattage, 35, 48

Whey protein, **98–99,** 216
Workouts
    calendar, 199
    description of CPE, 105–14
    nutrition for training days,
        86–87
    planning, 108
    power day
        description of workout,
            109–10
        level 1, 200, **200–201**
        level 2, 202, **202–3**
    progressions, 106–7
    regeneration day
        description of workout,
            113–14
        flexibility, **210–11**
        general regeneration,
            208–9
        hip pain, **212–13**
        knee pain, **212–13**
        lower back pain, **210–11**
        self-massage, **208–9**
        shin pain, **212–13**
        upper back/shoulder pain,
            210–11
    strength day
        description of workout,
            110–13
        level 1, 204, **204–5**
        level 2, 206, **206–7**
    work-to-regeneration ratio
        (2-to-1), 108

Y
Yogurt, 91, 216
Ys
    bent-over, 146–47, **146–47**
    floor, 140, **140**

ABOUT THE AUTHORS

Mark Verstegen is recognized as one of the world's most innovative sports performance experts. As the owner of the Athletes' Performance Institutes—cutting-edge training centers in Tempe, Arizona; Carson, California; and Las Vegas—he directs teams of performance specialists and nutritionists to train some of the biggest names in sports.

By teaching an integrated lifestyle and training program that blends strength, speed, flexibility, joint and "core" stability, and mental toughness, Verstegen helps athletes become not only faster and stronger but also more powerful, flexible, and resistant to injury and long-term back, hip, and other joint problems.

Because of his innovative techniques and up-to-date knowledge of sports performance, Verstegen is a sought-after consultant. He serves as director of performance for the NFL Players Association, is an advisor to Adidas, EAS, Gatorade, Keiser, Power Plate, and other leading performance-oriented companies, and serves as a consultant to numerous athletic governing bodies.

A dynamic speaker, Verstegen travels the world to address groups such as the American College of Sports Medicine, the National Strength and Conditioning Association, and many corporate audiences.

Verstegen and his training methods have been profiled by hundreds of national media outlets. He's a contributing columnist to *Men's Health* magazine. His first book, *Core Performance: The Revolutionary Workout Program to Transform Your Body and Your Life,* was published by Rodale in 2004. His most recent book, *Core Performance*

Essentials, was published by Rodale in 2006.

Verstegen began his coaching career at his alma mater, Washington State University. He served as assistant director of player development at Georgia Tech and in 1994 created the International Performance Institute on the campus of the IMG Sports Academy in Bradenton, Florida. In 1999, he moved to Phoenix to build the Athletes' Performance Institute, which quickly became the industry leader for training world-class athletes.

Verstegen and his wife, Amy, live in Scottsdale, Arizona.

Pete Williams is a veteran journalist who has written about sports, business, and fitness for numerous publications, including *USA Today, Men's Health,* and Street & Smith's *SportsBusiness Journal.* He is the author or coauthor of seven books, including the Rodale titles *Core Performance* and *Core Performance Essentials* (with Mark Verstegen),

and *Fun Is Good* (with Mike Veeck). Williams' most recent book is *The Draft: A Year inside the NFL's Search for Talent.* A graduate of the University of Virginia, he lives in the Tampa Bay, Florida, area with his wife, Suzy, and their two sons, and hosts *The Fitness Buff* radio show on WTAN AM 1340. His Web sites are www.petewilliams.net and www.fitnessbuffshow.com.

For more information on Mark Verstegen's Core training programs, including interactive workouts and nutritional information, please visit www.coreperformance.com/endurance. The site also offer sport-specific, DVD programs for tennis, golf, soccer, baseball, football, and other sports, along with Core training equipment and information on how to attend seminars and personalized training weeks at the Athletes' Performance Institutes in Tempe, Arizona; Carson, California; and Las Vegas.

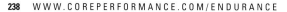